D0117183

ATI TEAS STUDY GUIDE
VERSION 6

TEAS 6 Test Prep and Practice Test
Questions for the Test of Essential
Academic Skills, Sixth Edition

TABLE OF CONTENTS

INTRODUCTION   i

1 PART I: READING   1

   ◆ Interpreting Text   3

   ◆ Graphic Representations   29
      of Information

2 PART II: MATHEMATICS   39

   ◆ Numbers And Operations   41

   ◆ Algebra   59

   ◆ Geometry and Measurement   67

3 PART III: SCIENCE   81

   ◆ Anatomy and Physiology   83

   ◆ Life Science   111

   ◆ Physical Science   125

   ◆ Scientific Reasoning   153

4 PART IV: ENGLISH AND   159
   LANGUAGE USE

   ◆ Grammar   161

   ◆ Vocabulary   185

5 PART V: TEST YOUR   197
   KNOWLEDGE

   ◆ Practice Test One   199

   ◆ Practice Test Two   241

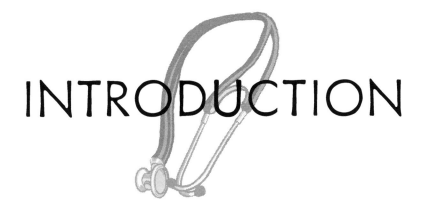

INTRODUCTION

The Test of Essential Academic Skills (TEAS) VI is a part of the admissions process for nursing and allied health programs around the country. Schools use the test to assess applicants' capabilities in four subject areas: reading, mathematics, science, and English and language usage. This guide will allow you to review your knowledge in these subject areas, apply your knowledge, and answer test questions.

What Is on the TEAS VI?

There are over 170 multiple-choice questions on the TEAS, 150 of which will be scored. The remaining twenty questions are unscored pretest questions that will not be indicated on the test. The number of questions for each subject area and subarea is indicated in the following table.

What Is on the TEAS VI?

Subject	SubAreas (scored questions)	Time Limit
Reading 53 questions: paragraph and passage comprehension and informational source comprehension	Key ideas and details (22) Craft and structure (14) Integration of knowledge and ideas (11)	64 minutes
Mathematics 36 questions: numbers and operations, measurement, data interpretation, and algebra	Numbers and algebra (23) Measurement and data (9)	54 minutes
Science 53 questions: scientific reasoning, human body science, life science, Earth science, and physical science	Human anatomy and physiology (32) Life and physical sciences (8) Scientific reasoning (7)	63 minutes
English and language usage 28 questions: grammar, punctuation, spelling, word meaning, and sentence structure	Conventions of standard English (9) Knowledge of language (9) Vocabulary acquisitions (6)	28 minutes
Total: 170 questions	150 scored questions	3 hours and 29 minutes

Scoring

You cannot pass or fail the TEAS VI exam. Instead, you will receive a score report that details the number of questions you got right in each section and also gives your percentile rank, which shows how you did in comparison to other test takers. Each school has its own entrance requirements, so be sure to check the requirements of the institutions you want to attend so that you can set appropriate goals for yourself. If you choose the computerized version of the test, you will receive your score immediately after testing.

How Is the Exam Administered?

The TEAS VI is administered by the Assessment Technologies Institute (ATI) at testing centers nationwide. To register for the TEAS, refer to the ATI website. You may choose to take a pencil-and-paper or computerized test. Both test types contain the same information and number of questions. You are encouraged the take the test in the format that is most comfortable for you.

On the day of your test, arrive early and be sure to bring proper identification, two No. 2 pencils, and your ATI login information. You are required to put away all personal belongings before the test begins. Cell phones and other electronic, photographic, recording, or listening devices are not permitted in the testing center at all. Calculators will be provided by the testing center. You will be permitted a ten-minute break after the mathematics section. For details on what to expect on test day, refer to the ATI website.

How to Use This Guide

The chapters in this book are divided into a review of the topics covered on the exam. This is not intended to teach you everything you'll see on the test: there is no way to cram all of that material into one book! Instead, we are going to help you recall information that you've already learned, and even more importantly, we'll show you how to apply that knowledge. Each chapter includes an extensive review with practice questions at the end to test your knowledge. With time, practice, and determination, you'll be well-prepared for test day.

This guide will help you master the most important test topics and also develop critical test-taking skills. To support this effort, the guide provides:

- ◆ organized concepts with detailed explanations
- ◆ practice questions with worked-through solutions
- ◆ key test-taking strategies
- ◆ simulated one-on-one tutor experience
- ◆ tips, tricks, and test secrets

About Accepted, Inc.

Accepted, Inc. uses industry professionals with decades' worth of knowledge in their fields, proven with degrees and honors in law, medicine, business, education, the military, and more, to produce high-quality test prep books for students.

Our study guides are specifically designed to increase any student's score, regardless of his or her current skill level. Our books are also shorter and more concise than typical study guides, so you can increase your score while significantly decreasing your study time.

We Want to Hear from You

Here at Accepted, Inc. our hope is that we not only taught you the relevant information needed to pass the exam, but that we helped you exceed all previous expectations. Our goal is to keep our guides concise, show you a few test tricks along the way, and ultimately help you succeed in your goals.

On that note, we are always interested in your feedback. To let us know if we've truly prepared you for the exam, please email us at support@acceptedinc.com. Feel free to include your test score!

Your success is our success. Good luck on the exam and in your future ventures.

Sincerely,

– The Accepted, Inc. Team –

PART I: READING

The TEAS VI Reading test includes questions about a wide range of media, including fiction and nonfiction passages, diagrams, graphs, sets of directions, and professional communications like emails and memos. Generally, these questions fall into three categories.

KEY IDEAS AND DETAILS questions test your comprehension of the text on a broad level. You will need to see the text as a whole, identify the main ideas, and explain how they lead to specific inferences and conclusions. You will also need to be able to discern the overall theme of a text and summarize it accurately.

CRAFT AND STRUCTURE questions test your understanding of the craft of writing. You might see questions about the use of language, point of view, and organization. You will need to be able to analyze the details of the passage and relate them to the overall organization and meaning of the passage.

INTEGRATION OF KNOWLEDGE questions ask you to incorporate your skills from the other categories to answer complex questions. Questions might ask you to evaluate a text, compare multiple texts, or examine other kinds of texts, such as visual media. In order to answer questions like this, you will need to synthesize the skills applied to other types of questions and go beyond analyzing texts to evaluating and judging them.

INTERPRETING TEXT

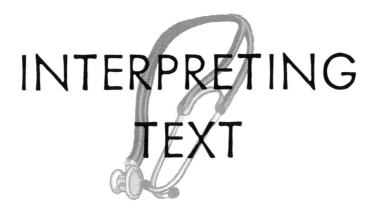

The Main Idea

The **MAIN IDEA** of a text describes the author's main topic and general perspective on that topic. It is expressed within and throughout the text. The reader can recognize the main idea in any text by considering the main topic and how it is addressed throughout the passage. On this test, you will be asked not only to identify the main idea of a text, but to differentiate it from the topic and theme and to summarize it clearly and concisely.

The main idea is closely connected to topic sentences and how they are supported in a text. Questions about the main idea may also deal with finding topic sentences, summarizing ideas in the text, or finding the supporting details of a text. In the sections that follow, determine the distinctions between all of these aspects of text and practice answering questions related to them.

Identifying the Main Idea

To identify the main idea, first identify the **TOPIC**. The difference between the two is simple. The **TOPIC** is the overall subject matter of the passage; the **MAIN IDEA** is what the author wants to say about that topic. The main idea covers the author's direct perspective about a topic, as distinct from the **THEME**, which is a generally true idea that the reader might derive from a text. Most of the time, a fiction text will have a theme, while a nonfiction text will have a main idea. This is true because in a nonfiction text, the author speaks more directly about a topic to the audience—his or her perspective is more apparent. For example, examine the following passage. As you read, think about the topic and what the author wants to communicate about that topic.

To determine the topic, ask yourself what you're reading about. To determine the main idea, ask yourself how the author feels about that topic.

The "shark mania" of recent years can be largely pinned on the sensationalistic media surrounding the animals: from the release of *Jaws* in 1975 to the week of ultra-hyped shark feeding frenzies and "worst shark attacks" countdowns known as *Shark Week*, popular culture both demonizes and fetishizes sharks until the public cannot get enough. Swimmers and beachgoers may look nervously for the telltale fin skimming the surface, but the reality is that shark bites are extremely rare and almost never unprovoked. Sharks attack people at very predictable times and for very predictable reasons: rough surf, poor visibility, or a swimmer sending visual and physical signals that mimic a shark's normal prey are just a few examples.

Of course, some places are just more dangerous for swimming. Shark attack "hot spots," such as the coasts of Florida, South Africa, and New Zealand, try a variety of solutions to protect tourists and surfers. Some beaches employ "shark nets" meant to keep sharks away from the beach, though these are controversial because they frequently trap other forms of marine life as well. Other beaches use spotters in helicopters and boats to alert beach officials when there are sharks in the area. In addition, there is an array of products that claim to offer personal protection from sharks, ranging from wetsuits in different colors to devices that broadcast electrical signals in an attempt to confuse the sharks' sensory organs. At the end of the day, though, beaches like these remain dangerous, and swimmers must assume the risk every time they paddle out from shore.

The author of this passage has a clear topic: sharks and the relationship between humans and sharks. In order to identify the main idea of the passage, ask yourself what the author wants to say about this topic. What does she or he want the reader to think or understand after reading? The author makes sure to provide information about several different aspects of the relationship between sharks and humans, and it is clear that she or he wishes to point out that humans must respect sharks as dangerous marine animals without sensationalizing the risk of attack.

Analyzing details the author includes and looking for similarities among them guides the reader to this conclusion. The passage describes sensationalistic media, then discusses how officials and governments try to protect beaches, and finally ends with the observation that people must ultimately take personal responsibility. By identifying these details, the author's main idea becomes clear.

Summarizing the main idea requires focusing on the connection between the different ideas and how that connection helps the reader draw a conclusion. A SUMMARY is a very brief restatement of the most important parts of an argument or text. To build a summary, start with the most important idea in a text. To continue building a longer summary, look for supporting details to add. Remember that when you summarize, your text should be much shorter than the original.

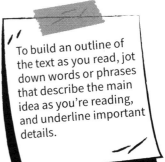

To build an outline of the text as you read, jot down words or phrases that describe the main idea as you're reading, and underline important details.

EXAMPLES

The art of the twentieth and twenty-first centuries demonstrates several aspects of modern societal advancement. A primary example is the advent and ascendancy of technology: new technologies have developed new avenues for art-making, and the globalization brought about by the Internet has simultaneously diversified the art world and brought it together. Even as artists are able to engage in a global conversation about the categories and characteristics of art, creating uniform understanding, artists have suddenly become able to express themselves in a diversity of ways for a diversity of audiences. The result has been a rapid change in the way art is made and consumed.

1. This passage is primarily concerned with
    A) the importance of art in the twenty-first century.
    B) using art to communicate overarching ideals to diverse communities.
    C) the importance of technology to art criticism.
    D) change in the understanding and creation of art in the modern period.

    D) is correct. The passage focuses on how the art of the modern period reflects the new technology and globalization made possible by the Internet.

2. Which of the following best describes the main idea of the passage?
    A) Modern advances in technology have diversified art-making and connected artists to distant places and ideas.
    B) Diversity in modern art is making it harder for art-viewers to understand and talk about that art.
    C) The use of technology to discuss art allows us to create standards for what art should be.
    D) Art-making before the invention of technology such as the Internet was disorganized and poorly understood.

A) is correct. According to the text, technology and the Internet have "simultaneously diversified the art world and brought it together."

Topic and Summary Sentences

Part of identifying the main idea is understanding the structure of a piece of writing. When looking at a short passage of one or two paragraphs, identifying the topic sentences and summary sentences will quickly tell the reader what the paragraphs are about and what conclusions the author wants the reader to draw. These sentences function as bookends to a paragraph or passage, telling readers what to think and then keeping the paragraph tightly tied together. The TOPIC SENTENCE is generally the first sentence or very near the first sentence in the paragraph. It introduces the reader to the topic by making a general statement about that topic, clearly and specifically directing the reader to access any previous experiences with that topic.

The SUMMARY SENTENCE of a paragraph, on the other hand, frequently (but not always!) comes at the end of a paragraph or passage, because it wraps up all of the ideas the passage presents. This sentence gives the reader an understanding of what the author wants to say about the topic and what conclusions can be drawn about it. While the topic sentence acts as an introduction to the topic, allowing the reader to activate his/her own ideas and experiences with the topic, the summary statement asks the reader to accept the author's ideas about that topic. Because of this, finding a summary sentence will help to quickly identify the main idea.

EXAMPLES

Altogether, Egypt is a land of tranquil monotony. The eye commonly travels either over a waste of waters, or over a green plain unbroken by elevations. The hills which enclose the Nile valley have level tops, and sides that are bare of trees, or shrubs, or flowers, or even mosses. The sky is generally cloudless. No fog or mist enwraps the distance in mystery; no rainstorm sweeps across the scene; no rainbow spans the empyrean; no shadows chase each other over the landscape. There is an entire absence of picturesque scenery. A single broad river, unbroken within the limits of Egypt even by a rapid, two flat strips of green plain at its side, two low lines of straight-topped hills beyond them, and a boundless open space where the river divides itself into half a dozen sluggish branches before reaching the sea, constitute Egypt, which is by nature a southern Holland—"weary, stale, flat and unprofitable."

George Rawlinson, *Ancient Egypt*, 1886

1. Which of the following statements is the topic sentence?

   A) *There is an entire absence of picturesque scenery.*

   B) *Altogether, Egypt is a land of tranquil monotony.*

   C) *The sky is generally cloudless.*

   D) *A single broad river, unbroken within the limits of Egypt even by a rapid, two flat strips of green plain at its side, two low lines of straight-topped hills beyond them, and a boundless open space where the river divides itself into half a dozen sluggish branches before reaching the sea, constitute Egypt, which is by nature a southern Holland—weary, stale, flat and unprofitable.*

   B) is correct. It introduces the topic of the paragraph (Egypt) and makes a general statement that is supported by later details.

2. Which of the following best states what the author wants the reader to understand after reading the summary sentence?

   A) There isn't much to get excited about while visiting Egypt.

   B) Egypt is a poverty-stricken wasteland.

   C) The land of Egypt is worn out from overuse.

   D) The land of Egypt lacks anything fresh or inspiring.

   D) is correct. The words *worn*, *stale* and *unprofitable* suggest a lack of freshness or anything that stimulates enthusiasm.

Supporting Details

Between a topic sentence and a summary sentence, the rest of a paragraph is built by supporting details. Supporting details can come in many forms; the purpose of the passage dictates the type of information that will be used to support the main idea. A persuasive passage may use specific facts and data, or it may detail specific reasons for the author's opinion. An informative passage will primarily use facts about the topic to support the main idea. Even a narrative passage will have supporting details—the specific things the author says to develop the story and characters.

The most important aspect of supporting details is exactly what the name says: they must support the main idea. Looking at the various supporting details and how they work with one another will solidify an understanding of the author's perspective on a topic and what the main idea of the passage really is. The supporting details contain important information key to understanding the passage.

Identifying Supporting Details

How can a reader identify the most important pieces of information in a passage? SUPPORTING DETAILS build the argument and contain the key ideas upon which the main idea rests. While finding the supporting details will help reveal the main idea, it is actually easier to find the most important supporting details by understanding the main idea first; then the pieces that make up the argument will become clear.

SIGNAL WORDS or transitions and conjunctions that explain to the reader how one sentence or idea is connected to another hint at supporting ideas. These words and phrases can be anywhere in a sentence, and it is important to understand what each signal word means. Signal words can add information, provide counterarguments, create organization in the passage, or draw conclusions. Some common signal words and terms include *for example*, *in particular*, *in addition*, *besides*, *in contrast*, *therefore*, *because*, or many other similar phrases.

EXAMPLES

The war is inevitable—and let it come! I repeat it, sir, let it come! It is in vain, sir, to extenuate the matter. Gentlemen may cry, "Peace! Peace!"—but there is no peace. The war is actually begun! The next gale that sweeps from the north will bring to our ears the clash of resounding arms! Our brethren are already in the field! Why stand we here idle? What is it that gentlemen wish? What would they have? Is life so dear, or peace so sweet, as to be purchased at the price of chains and slavery? Forbid it, Almighty God! I know not what course others may take; but as for me, give me liberty, or give me death!

Patrick Henry, "The Speech to the Virginia Convention," 1775

1. In the third line of the text, the word *but* signals which of the following?

   A) an example

   B) a consequence

   C) a reason

   D) a counterargument

   D) is correct. The argument or claim that the country should be at peace precedes the word *but*. *But* introduces the counterargument that peace is impossible; the war has begun.

Evaluating Supporting Details

Besides using supporting details to understand a main idea, the reader must evaluate them for relevance and consistency. An author selects supporting details that help organize the passage and support the main idea. Sometimes, the author's bias may cause him or her to omit details that do not directly support the main idea or that may even support an opposing idea. A reader must recognize not only what the author says, but also what the author leaves out.

To understand how a supporting detail relates to the main idea, a reader must first understand the purpose of the passage. What is the author trying to communicate? How does the author want the reader to respond? Every passage has a specific goal, and each paragraph in a passage is meant to support that goal. For each supporting detail, the position in the text, the signal words, and the specific content work together to alert the reader to the relationship between the supporting ideas and the main ideas.

Close reading of a text requires taking note of its striking features. For example, does a point in the text appeal to your sense of justice? Does a description seem rather exaggerated or overstated? Do certain words seem emotive, like *agonizing*? Are rhetorical questions being used to lead you to a certain conclusion?

In general, an author includes details that support the main idea; however, the reader must decide how those ideas relate to one another and uncover any weaknesses in their support of the author's argument. This is particularly important in a persuasive piece of writing, when an author may display bias in his or her choice of supporting details. Discovering the author's bias and how the supporting details reveal that bias is key to understanding a text.

EXAMPLES

In England in the fifties came the Crimean War, with the deep stirring of national feeling which accompanied it, and the passion of gratitude and admiration which was poured forth on Miss Florence Nightingale for her work on behalf of our wounded soldiers. It was universally felt that there was work for women, even in war—the work of cleansing, setting in order, breaking down red tape, and soothing the vast sum of human suffering which every war is bound to cause. Miss Nightingale's work in war was work that never had been done until women came forward to do it, and her message to her countrywomen was educate yourselves, prepare, make ready; never imagine that your task can be done by instinct, without training and preparation. Painstaking study, she insisted, was just as necessary as a preparation for women's work as for men's work; and she bestowed the whole of the monetary gift offered her by the gratitude of the nation to form training-schools for nurses at St. Thomas's and King's College Hospitals.

Millicent Garrett Fawcett, *Women's Suffrage: A Short History of a Great Movement*, 1888

1. Which of the following best states the bias of the passage?

   A) Society underestimates the capacity of women.

   B) Generally, women are not prepared to make substantial contributions to society.

   C) If women want power, they need to prove themselves.

   D) One strong woman cannot represent all women.

   A) is correct. The author suggests that Florence Nightingale was the first person to undertake humanitarian work on the battlefield. As a female pioneer, Nightingale proved that women were capable of challenging responsibilities and making major contributions to society.

2. Which of the following best summarizes what the author left out of the passage?

   A) Women can fight in wars.

   B) Other women should be recognized.

   C) Women need to stop wasting time giving speeches at conventions and start proving themselves.

   D) Without the contributions of women, society suffers.

   D) is correct. The author does emphasize that "Miss Nightingale's work in war was work that never had been done until women came forward to do it."

Facts and Opinions

Authors use both facts and opinions as supporting details. While it is usually a simple task to identify between the two, sometimes an author might mix facts and opinions in such a way that the two become convoluted; in addition, an author might state an opinion as if it is a fact. The difference between the two is simple: a FACT is a piece of information that can be verified as true or false by any person, and it retains the quality of truthfulness (or not) no matter who verifies it. On the other hand, an opinion expresses a belief held by the speaker and may or may not be something each audience member agrees with.

To distinguish between fact and opinion, ask if a statement can be proven. Look for subjectivity by asking if an observation could vary according to the situation or person observing.

EXAMPLES

I remember thinking how comfortable it was, this division of labor which made it unnecessary for me to study fogs, winds, tides, and navigation, in order to visit my friend who lived across an arm of the sea. It was good that men should be specialists, I mused. The peculiar knowledge of the pilot and captain sufficed for many thousands of people who knew no more of the sea and navigation than I knew. On the other hand, instead of having to devote my energy to the learning of a multitude of things, I concentrated it upon a few particular things, such as, for instance, the analysis of Poe's place in American literature—an essay of mine, by the way, in the current *Atlantic*. Coming aboard, as I passed through the cabin, I had noticed with greedy eyes a stout gentleman reading the *Atlantic*, which was open at my very essay. And there it was again, the division of labor, the special knowledge of the pilot and captain which permitted the stout gentleman to read my special knowledge on Poe while they carried him safely from Sausalito to San Francisco.

Jack London, *The Sea-Wolf*, 1904

1. Which of the following best summarizes an opinion stated by the narrator?

    A) Poe had a place in American literature.

    B) The narrator had no knowledge of the sea and navigation.

    C) Having specialized knowledge sets people apart and makes them superior.

    D) Division of labor is a beneficial practice.

    D) is correct. The narrator provides several facts proving his opinion that he and the other passengers benefit from the specialized knowledge and labor of others.

GO ON

Text Structure

The structure of a text determines how the reader understands the argument and how various details interact to form the argument. There are many ways to arrange text, and varying types of arrangements have distinct characteristics. Specific text structures include:

- cause and effect: the author describes a situation and then its effects
- compare and contrast: the author explores the similarities and differences between two or more things
- problem and solution: the author presents a problem and offers a solution
- descriptive: the author describes a topic
- chronological: the author lists events in the order in which they happened

To identify the organizing structure of a passage, look at the order in which the author presents information and the transitions used to connect those pieces. Structures such as problem-solution or cause-effect will use transitions that show causal relationships: *because, as a result, consequently, therefore.* These structures might also use transitions that show contradiction (*however, alternatively, although*). The former may provide solutions, while the latter can explain alternative causes.

When analyzing a text, a reader should consider how text structure impacts the author's meaning. Most important, readers must be aware of how an author presents information in order to emphasize an idea. For example, including a contrasting idea makes a central idea stand out, or including a series of concrete examples strongly supports an argument.

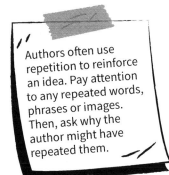

Authors often use repetition to reinforce an idea. Pay attention to any repeated words, phrases or images. Then, ask why the author might have repeated them.

EXAMPLES

It was the green heart of the canyon, where the walls swerved back from the rigid plan and relieved their harshness of line by making a little sheltered nook and filling it to the brim with sweetness and roundness and softness. Here all things rested. Even the narrow stream ceased its turbulent down-rush long enough to form a quiet pool. On one side, beginning at the very lip of the pool, was a tiny meadow, a cool, resilient surface of green that extended to the base of the frowning wall. Beyond the pool a gentle slope of earth ran up and up to meet the opposing wall. Fine grass covered the slope—grass that was spangled with flowers, with here and there patches of color, orange and purple and golden. Below, the canyon was shut in. There was no view. The walls leaned together abruptly and the canyon ended in a chaos of rocks, moss-covered and hidden by a green screen of vines and creepers and boughs of trees. Up the canyon rose far hills and peaks, the big foothills, pine-covered and remote. And far beyond, like clouds upon the border of the slay, towered minarets of white, where the Sierra's eternal snows flashed austerely the blazes of the sun.

Jack London, "All Gold Canyon," 1905

1. Which of the following best describes the structure of this text?

   A) order of importance

   B) cause and effect

   C) problem and solution

   D) spatial

   D) is correct. The description of the nook begins with a general impression, moves from one side to the area beyond the pool, to below the heart of the canyon, and finally to what is above the canyon.

2. How does the text structure emphasize the central idea of the passage?

   A) The logical reasons for needing to rest while hiking make the author's argument compelling.

   B) By explaining the activities within the canyon, the author convinces the reader that the canyon is safe.

   C) By describing the area to the side, below, and above the canyon, the author is able to emphasize the softness of the heart of the canyon.

   D) The concrete examples that are included in the passage demonstrate the author's view that beauty is found in nature.

Drawing Conclusions

Reading text begins with making sense of the explicit meanings of information or a narrative. Understanding text occurs as readers draw conclusions and make logical inferences from a text. To draw a CONCLUSION, readers must first consider the details or facts. Then, they arrive at a conclusion from these details; the conclusion is the next logical point in the thought sequence. For example, in a Hemingway story, an old man is sitting alone in a café. The young waiter says that the café is closing, but the old man continues to drink. The waiter starts closing up, and the old man signals for a refill. Based on these details, the reader might conclude that the old man has not understood the young waiter's desire for him to leave.

An INFERENCE is distinct from a conclusion. An inference is an educated guess that readers take based on details in the text as well as their own knowledge; it is information that enriches the reader's understanding of the literal meaning of the text. Readers use their own knowledge when considering what the author suggests through the details offered in descriptions of decisions or situations. Returning to the Hemingway story about the old man, the reader might infer that the old man is lonely, enjoys being in the café, and is reluctant to leave.

When reading fictional text, inferring character motivations is essential. The actions of the characters move the plot forward; understanding the meaning of the series of events requires making sense of the characters' reasoning for their actions. Hemingway includes contrasting details as the young waiter and an older waiter discuss the old man. The older waiter sympathizes with the old man because this waiter, too, needs a light for the night; both old men are lonely and experience a sense of emptiness in life, which motivates them to seek out the café.

Readers must also be able to connect texts to each other. A reader should recognize that the Hemingway story about the old man in the café, for instance, shares similarities with other Hemingway stories about individuals struggling to deal with loss and loneliness in a dignified way. Readers can even integrate their own personal connections and experiences into their reading. When readers read persuasive texts, for instance, they may connect the arguments in those texts to counterarguments and opposing evidence of which they are aware. They use these connections to infer meaning.

Considering a character's motivations means asking: *What does the character want to achieve? What will the character get by accomplishing this? What does the character seem to value the most?*

EXAMPLE

I believe it is difficult for those who publish their own memoirs to escape the imputation of vanity; nor is this the only disadvantage under which they labor: it is also their misfortune, that what is uncommon is rarely, if ever, believed, and what is obvious we are apt to turn from with disgust, and to charge the writer with impertinence. People generally think those memoirs only worthy to be read or remembered which abound in great or striking events, those, in short, which in a high degree excite either admiration or pity: all others they consign to contempt and oblivion. It is therefore, I confess, not a little hazardous in a private and obscure individual, and a stranger too, thus to solicit the indulgent attention of the public; especially when I own I offer here the history of neither a saint, a hero, nor a tyrant. I believe there are few events in my life, which have not happened to many: it is true the incidents of it are numerous; and, did I consider myself an European, I might say my sufferings were great: but when I compare my lot with that of most of my countrymen, I regard myself as a *particular favorite of Heaven*, and acknowledge the mercies of Providence in every occurrence of my life. If then the following narrative does not appear sufficiently interesting to engage general attention, let my motive be some excuse for its publication. I am not so foolishly vain as to expect from it either immortality or literary reputation. If it affords any satisfaction to my numerous friends, at whose request it has been written, or in the smallest degree promotes the interests of humanity, the ends for which it was undertaken will be fully attained, and every wish of my heart gratified. Let it therefore be remembered, that, in wishing to avoid censure, I do not aspire to praise.

Olaudah Equiano, *The Interesting Narrative of the Life of Olaudah Equiano, The African, Written by Himself*, 1789

Which of the following best explains the primary motivation of the narrator?

A) He wants his audience to know that he is not telling his story out of vanity.

B) The narrator is hoping that people will praise his courage.

C) The narrator is honoring the wishes of his friends.

D) He is hoping that people will be influenced by his story and the human condition will improve.

D) is correct. "In the smallest degree promotes the interests of humanity, the ends for which it was undertaken will be fully attained, and every wish of my heart gratified." The narrator's use of the word humanity could mean he wants to improve the human condition or that he wants to increase human benevolence and brotherly love.

Understanding the Author

It is important to approach every passage with the understanding that an author chooses words, structures, and content with specific purpose and intent. Without that assumption, it will be impossible to understand the author. With that assumption, a reader can discern why an author uses those words and structures and how they relate to the content.

The Author's Purpose

The author of a passage sets out to communicate a specific idea to an audience with a specific goal in mind. The AUTHOR'S PURPOSE is expressed by determining why an author wants a reader to understand the main idea. There are four basic purposes to which an author can write; within each of these general purposes, the author may also direct the audience to take a clear action or respond in a certain way.

The purpose for which an author writes a passage is also connected to the structure of that text. In a NARRATIVE, the author tells the reader a story, often to illustrate a theme or idea the reader needs to consider. In a narrative, the author will use the characteristics of storytelling, such as chronological order, characters, and a defined setting. Identifying these characteristics in a text should indicate that the author wishes to communicate a theme or main idea stemming from the events or characters in the story.

In an EXPOSITORY passage, on the other hand, the author simply explains an idea or topic to the reader. The main idea will probably be a factual statement or a direct assertion of a broadly held opinion. Expository writing can come in many forms, but one essential feature is a fair and balanced representation of a topic: the author may explore one detailed aspect or a broad range of characteristics, but he or she intends mainly to present the details or ideas to the reader to make a decision.

Similarly, in TECHNICAL writing, the author's purpose is to explain specific processes, techniques, or equipment in order for the reader to use that process or equipment to obtain the desired result. In this writing, look for chronological or spatial organization, specialized vocabulary, and imperative or directive structures.

The categories of writing discussed above mostly communicate information to a reader so that he or she can take action or make a decision. In contrast, in PERSUASIVE writing, the author actively sets out to convince the reader to accept an opinion or belief.

Much like expository writing, persuasive writing can take many organizational forms; however specific techniques, or RHETORICAL

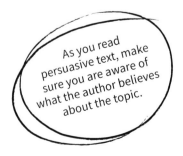

As you read persuasive text, make sure you are aware of what the author believes about the topic.

STRATEGIES, assist the author in building an argument. Readers can identify these strategies in order to clearly understand what an author wants them to believe, how the author's perspective and purpose may lead to bias, and whether the passage includes any logical fallacies. Common rhetorical strategies include the appeals to logos, ethos, and pathos. An author uses these to build trust with the reader, explain the logical points of an argument, and convince the reader of the author's opinion.

An ETHOS or ETHICAL APPEAL uses balanced, fair language and seeks to build a trusting relationship between the author and the reader. An author might explain his or her credentials, include the reader in an argument, or offer concessions to an opposing argument. LOGOS, LOGICAL APPEAL, builds on that trust by providing facts and support for the author's opinion, explaining the argument with clear connections and reasoning. At this point, the reader should beware of logical fallacies that falsely connect unrelated ideas and build arguments on incorrect premises.

Finally, an author convinces the reader to accept an opinion or belief by demonstrating that not only is it the most logical option, but it also appeals to his or her emotional reaction to a topic. PATHOS, the APPEAL TO EMOTION, does not depend on reasonable connections between ideas; rather, it reminds a reader through imagery, strong language, and personal connections that the author's argument aligns with the reader's best interests. Many persuasive passages use all three rhetorical strategies to best appeal to a reader.

EXAMPLES

Evident truth. Made so plain by our good Father in Heaven, that all feel and understand it, even down to brutes and creeping insects. The ant, who has toiled and dragged a crumb to his nest, will furiously defend the fruit of his labor, against whatever robber assails him. So plain, that the most dumb and stupid slave that ever toiled for a master, does constantly know that he is wronged. So plain that no one, high or low, ever does mistake it, except in a plainly selfish way; for although volume upon volume is written to prove slavery a very good thing, we never hear of the man who wishes to take the good of it, by being a slave himself.

Most governments have been based, practically, on the denial of the equal rights of men, as I have, in part, stated them; ours began, by affirming those rights. They said, some men are too ignorant, and vicious, to share in government. Possibly so, said we; and, by your system, you would always keep them ignorant and vicious. We proposed to give all a chance; and we expected the weak to grow stronger, the ignorant, wiser; and all better, and happier together.

We made the experiment; and the fruit is before us. Look at it. Think of it. Look at it, in its aggregate grandeur, of extent of country, and numbers of population, of ship, and steamboat, and rail...

Abraham Lincoln, 1858

1. The author's purpose is to

   A) explain ideas.

   B) narrate a story.

   C) describe a situation.

   D) persuade the reader to accept an idea.

   D) is correct. The author is providing logical reasons and evidence that slavery is wrong, that it violates the American belief in equal rights.

2. To achieve his purpose, the author primarily uses

   A) concrete analogies.

   B) logical reasoning.

   C) emotional appeals.

   D) images.

   B) is correct. The author uses logic when he points out that one who claims that slavery is good never "wishes to take the good of it, by being a slave..." The author also points out that the principle of the United States is to give everyone, including the "ignorant," opportunity; then, he challenges his listeners to look at the fruit of this principle, saying, "Look at it, in its aggregate grandeur, of extent of country, and numbers of population, of ship, and steamboat..."

The Audience

The structure, purpose, main idea, and language of a text all converge on one target: the intended audience. An author makes decisions about every aspect of a piece of writing based on that audience, and a reader can evaluate the writing through the lens of that audience. By considering the probable reactions of an intended audience, readers can determine many things: whether or not they are part of that intended audience, the author's purpose for using specific techniques or devices, the biases of the author and how they appear in the writing, and how the author uses rhetorical strategies. While a reader can evaluate each of these separately, identifying and considering the intended audience deepens the understanding of a text and highlights its details.

To identify the intended audience, consider several aspects of the text. First of all, look at the main idea and/or theme of the passage. Who is most likely to care about that idea, benefit from it, or need to know about the topic? If the text is persuasive, who is the author trying to persuade? If it's explanatory, who would benefit from having this knowledge?

Next, in order to refine your understanding of an audience, look at the language. An author tailors the language in a passage to appeal to the intended audience, so the reader can study the language to better understand the audience. Formal language is used to appeal to academics or people in a professional setting, while media like commercials and blogs will use more informal language to reach a wider audience. For example, employees use different language when writing emails to the boss than in emails to coworkers.

On the TEAS you're likely to see text from items like memos, emails, and print media. Identifying the audience for these items will help in answering questions about them. A brochure meant for a public bulletin board is likely to have a specific purpose and tone, as would a job application, a letter to a colleague, or a company-wide announcement. Use your knowledge of the audience to assess the text's main idea, tone, and structure.

EXAMPLE

Date: April 6, 2016

Title: End of School Cleaning Policy

The janitorial staff will begin cleaning classrooms in preparation for summer classes on June 16, 2016. For this reason, teachers are required to have their classrooms emptied of all personal effects by end of day on June 15, 2016. Any personal effects left behind will be placed in storage until claimed by the owner.

1. The author of this memo was most likely which of the following?

   A) a teacher

   B) a school administrator

   C) a student

   D) a member of the janitorial staff

   B) is correct. The tone of the memo is formal and makes specific demands of the teachers, meaning it was likely written by someone in a position of authority, such as a school administrator.

Tone and Mood

One important aspect of communication between author and audience occurs subtly, through the tone and mood developed throughout a passage. The TONE describes the author's attitude toward the topic, distinct from the MOOD, which is the pervasive feeling or atmosphere in a passage that provokes specific emotions in the reader. The importance of the distinction between these two aspects of text lies once again in the audience: the mood influences a reader's emotional state in the piece, while the tone establishes the relationship between the audience and the author. Does the author intend to instruct the audience? Is the author more experienced than the audience, or does she or he wish to establish a friendly or equal relationship? In each of these cases, the author can use a different tone to establish the appropriate level of communication.

To determine mood and tone in a passage, look primarily to the DICTION, or word choice of the author. Many readers make the mistake of thinking about the ideas an author puts forth and using those alone to determine tone; a much better practice is to separate specific words from the text and look for patterns in connotation and emotion. By considering categories of words used by the author, a reader can determine both the overall emotional atmosphere of a text and the attitude of an author toward the subject.

Every word has not only a literal meaning, but also a CONNOTATIVE MEANING that relies on the common emotions, associations, and experiences an audience might associate with that word. Consider the following words that are all synonyms: *dog, puppy, cur, mutt, canine, pet*. Two of these words, *dog* and *canine*, are neutral words, without strong associations or emotions. Two others, *pet* and *puppy*, have positive associations, and the last two, *cur* and *mutt*, have negative associations. A passage that uses one pair of these words versus another pair activates the positive or negative reactions of the audience.

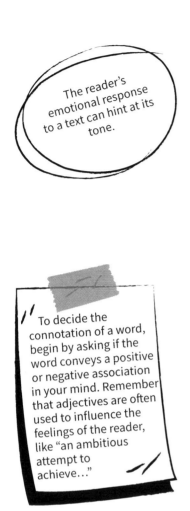

The reader's emotional response to a text can hint at its tone.

To decide the connotation of a word, begin by asking if the word conveys a positive or negative association in your mind. Remember that adjectives are often used to influence the feelings of the reader, like "an ambitious attempt to achieve…"

EXAMPLES

Day had broken cold and grey, exceedingly cold and grey, when the man turned aside from the main Yukon trail and climbed the high earth-bank, where a dim and little-travelled trail led eastward through the fat spruce timberland. It was a steep bank, and he paused for breath at the top, excusing the act to himself by looking at his watch. It was nine o'clock. There was no sun nor hint of sun, though there was not a cloud in the sky. It was a clear day, and yet there seemed an intangible pall over the face of things, a subtle gloom that made the day dark, and that was due to the absence of sun. This fact did not worry the man. He was used to the lack of sun. It had been days since he had seen the sun, and he knew that a few more days must pass before that cheerful orb, due south, would just peep above the skyline and dip immediately from view.

Jack London, "To Build a Fire," 1908

1. Which of the following best describes the mood of the passage?

   A) exciting and adventurous

   B) fierce and determined

   C) bleak and forbidding

   D) grim, yet hopeful

   C) is correct. The man is oblivious to the gloom and darkness of the day that was *exceedingly cold and grey*.

2. Which of the following best describes the connotation of the word *pall*?

   A) a death-like covering

   B) a vague sense of familiarity

   C) an intimation of communal strength

   D) an understanding of the struggle ahead

   A) is correct. Within the context of the sentence, *It was a clear day, and yet there seemed an intangible pall over the face of things, a subtle gloom that made the day dark…* the words *gloom* and *dark* are suggestive of death; the phrase *over the face* suggests a covering.

Words in Context

The TEAS will ask you to determine the definition of words in context, meaning as they appear within the text. This can be a slightly more difficult task than simply knowing the basic definition of a word, as you may be required to analyze how the author is using the word in this specific text.

Context Clues

There are many different parts of a passage that can be helpful in determining meaning from context: the sentence the word appears in, specific words around the unfamiliar word, other words in the passage that reference the unfamiliar word, and the overall understanding of the passage, including main idea, mood, and tone.

To grasp the meaning of unfamiliar words, readers may use context clues or hints in the text. Using context clues is especially helpful for determining the appropriate meaning of a word with multiple definitions.

One type of context clue is a DEFINITION or DESCRIPTION CLUE. Sometimes, authors may use a difficult word; then say, "that is" or "which is" to signal the reader that they are providing a definition. An author may also provide a synonym or restate the idea in familiar words:

Readers should be attentive to signal words like *because, since, in contrast, instead of, therefore, however,* and *as a result*. These signal words indicate how an unfamiliar word is related to the overall meaning of the sentence or paragraph.

Teachers often prefer teaching students with <u>intrinsic</u> motivation; these students have an <u>internal</u> desire to learn.

The meaning of *intrinsic* is restated as *internal*.

Similarly, authors may include EXAMPLE CLUES by providing an example of the unfamiliar word close to the word:

Teachers may view extrinsic rewards as <u>efficacious</u>; however, an individual student may not be interested in what the teacher offers. For example, a student who is diabetic may not feel any incentive to work when offered a sweet treat.

Efficacious is explained with an example demonstrating the effectiveness (and lack thereof) of extrinsic rewards.

Another commonly used context clue is the CONTRAST/ANTONYM CLUE. In this case, authors indicate that the unfamiliar word is the opposite of a familiar word:

<u>In contrast</u> to <u>intrinsic</u> motivation, <u>extrinsic</u> motivation is contingent on teachers offering rewards that are appealing.

The phrase *in contrast* tells the reader that *extrinsic* is the opposite of *intrinsic*.

EXAMPLES

1. One challenge of teaching is finding ways to incentivize, or to motivate, learning.

   Which of the following is the meaning of *incentivize* as used in the sentence?

   A) encourage

   B) reward

   C) challenge

   D) improve

   A) is correct. The word *incentivize* is defined immediately with the synonym *motivate*, or encourage.

2. If an extrinsic reward is extremely desirable, a student may become so apprehensive he or she cannot focus. That is, the student may experience such intense pressure to perform the reward undermines its intent.

   Which of the following is the meaning of *apprehensive* as used in the sentence?

   A) uncertain

   B) distracted

   C) anxious

   D) forgetful

Figurative Language

FIGURES OF SPEECH are expressions that are understood to have a non-literal meaning. Instead of meaning what is actually said, figurative language suggests meaning by speaking of a subject as if it is something else. When Shakespeare says, "All the world's a stage, / And all men and women merely players," he isn't stating that the world is literally a stage. Instead, it functions like a stage, with men and women giving performances as if they were actors on a stage.

Figures of speech extend the meaning of words by giving readers a new way to think about the subject. Thinking of the world as a stage on which people are performing is a new way of thinking about life. After reading Shakespeare's metaphor, people may reflect on how often they play a role themselves: they may wonder when their behavior is genuine, if they are too worried about others evaluating their performance, and so on. Figures of speech engage a reader's imagination and add emphasis to different aspects of their subject.

A METAPHOR is essentially an analogy. It is figurative language that explains something unfamiliar—the topic—through a vehicle familiar to the reader, correlating the two to explain something to the reader or enhance an idea. The familiar vehicle helps the reader understand a new or unfamiliar topic. For example, if a person refers to a problem as "the elephant in the room," the topic is the problem; *elephant* is the vehicle expressing just how overwhelming and undeniable that problem is (as big and powerful as an elephant, though not literally one).

A SIMILE is figurative language that directly points to similarities between two things. The author is using a familiar vehicle to express an idea about the topic. For example, in his poem "The Rime of the Ancient Mariner" Samuel Taylor Coleridge describes his ship as "Idle as a painted ship upon a painted ocean." Readers have most likely seen a painting of a ship; Coleridge harnesses this knowledge not only to explain that the ship is still, but to emphasize just how motionless and quiet it really is.

> Similes usually use words such as *like* or *as* in phrasing; metaphors do not.

EXAMPLES

1. The coach was thrilled his team won their final game. The fact that his son scored the winning goal was just the icing on the cake.

    In the sentence, *icing on the cake* refers to which of the following?

A) an unfortunate occurrence

B) an added benefit

C) a surprise event

D) an accidental delight

B) is correct. The fact that the coach was already thrilled implies that the *icing on the cake* provides an extra level of enjoyment.

In shape Egypt is like a lily with a crooked stem. A broad blossom terminates it at its upper end; a button of a bud projects from the stalk a little below the blossom, on the left-hand side. The broad blossom is the Delta, extending a direct distance of a hundred and eighty miles, which the projection of the coast—the graceful swell of the petals—enlarges to two hundred and thirty. The bud is an oasis, a natural depression in the hills that shut in the Nile valley on the west, which has been rendered cultivable for many thousands of years. The long stalk of the lily is the Nile valley itself, which is a ravine scooped in the rocky soil for seven hundred miles to the apex of the Delta, sometimes not more than a mile broad, never more than eight or ten miles. No other country in the world is so strangely shaped, so long compared to its width, so straggling, so hard to govern from a single center.

George Rawlinson, *Ancient Egypt*, 1886

2. The author uses the simile *In shape Egypt is like a lily with a crooked stem* in order to emphasize which of the following?

A) the length of the Nile valley

B) the fertility of Egypt's soil

C) Egypt's beauty

D) the uniqueness of Egypt's shape

D) is correct. The image of Egypt as a long-stemmed flower emphasizes how unusual its shape is, as explained in the final sentence: *No other country in the world is so strangely shaped, so long compared to its width, so straggling, so hard to govern from a single center.*

Research Skills

Research is the process of searching for credible information, or sources. Sources take various forms, such as written documentation, audio-visual materials, information found over the Internet, in-person interviews, and more. Sources may answer specific questions posed in a text, enrich the information provided on a topic by the writer, or support a writer's argument. In the twenty-first century, locating sources is easy; however, finding and determining quality sources involves careful evaluation of each one. The TEAS

Reading test will include questions that ask you to categorize types of sources and evaluate which sources are appropriate for a specific task.

Evaluating Sources

It is best to begin evaluating sources by evaluating the credibility of the author. Consideration should be given to the motivation of the author: the author's purpose or reason for writing the text may indicate whether the text is biased. Next, researchers must identify the author's background and expertise. Although educational credentials are significant, firsthand experience offers equally reliable information.

Questions to consider include:

1. Is the source current?
2. If it is a secondary source, is it based on both primary as well as other secondary sources?
3. Is the author an expert in the area of study? Does he or she cite relevant information from other authorities on the topic?
4. Is the author's purpose clear? That is, is there any apparent bias?
5. What does the author assume is true?
6. Does the author present multiple viewpoints?
7. Does the content align with other reliable sources on the topic?

It can also be helpful to look at the place the text was published. Sources like academic journals and established newspapers are more likely to have rigorous standards for publication, which means their articles are fairly reliable. On the other hand, open-source platforms like blogs and websites are more likely to contain biased material.

To evaluate a website, determine who the intended audience is and if there's an agenda in terms of selling something or promoting a belief system. For example, a health website created by a company selling nutritional supplements will not be as authoritative as a site maintained by a government health organization, since it might omit relevant information that would hinder its sales. Similarly, a website for a particular candidate for public office might not be as good a source of unbiased policy information as a website maintained by a neutral nonprofit organization if elements or consequences of those policies do not align with the candidate's platform.

EXAMPLE

1. Which of the following sources is most appropriate for researching the health effects of smoking?

   A) the personal website of a local doctor

   B) a commercial produced by tobacco farming advocates

   C) a website run by the Centers for Disease Control

   D) a book titled *101 Ways to Quit Smoking*

   C) is correct. The Centers for Disease Control, as a government agency, will most likely offer the least biased information out of the four choices.

Types of Sources

The sources researchers use depend on their purpose. If the researcher's purpose is to analyze, interpret, or critique a historical event, a creative work, or a natural phenomenon, the researcher will use **PRIMARY** or original sources. Primary sources were produced by people with firsthand experience of an event. Examples of primary sources include:

- letters and emails
- autobiographies, diaries, and memoirs
- firsthand or eyewitness accounts or descriptions of events
- interviews, questionnaires, and surveys
- speeches and lectures
- photographs, drawings, and paintings
- news stories written at the time of the event

The written analysis or interpretation of a primary source is considered a **SECONDARY SOURCE**. These sources are written by people who did not have firsthand experience of the topic being described. Instead, authors of secondary sources examine primary sources in order to draw conclusions or make generalizations about people, events, and ideas. Examples of secondary sources include:

- literary criticism and interpretation
- biographies
- historical criticism
- political analyses
- essays on ethics and social policies

EXAMPLE

1. Which of the following is an example of a secondary source for an article on local highways?

   A) an online opinion column promoting tax incentives for those who carpool

   B) photographs of traffic accidents

   C) data from the city's transportation department

   D) an autobiography of a city official who led efforts to improve local infrastructure

   A) is correct. It describes a secondary source that analyzes a topic rather than presenting first-hand experience of it.

two

GRAPHIC REPRESENTATIONS OF INFORMATION

In addition to locating information in text passages, the TEAS also requires test takers to answer questions about a variety of figures, including maps, graphs and charts, illustrations, and advertisements. The TEAS will test your ability to use these graphic representations of information to answer similar questions to those asked about text passages. You'll be asked to:

♦ identify specific facts or patterns from the figure

♦ identify how the author uses specific features in the figure

♦ make connections between the figure and a related text passage

Maps

A MAP is a visual representation of space. It shows the relative location of a number of features, including roads, buildings, cities, and natural features like bodies of water and mountains. Many of these features will likely be represented by symbols. For example, a forested area might be marked with a drawing of a single tree, and railroad tracks might be indicated using a dotted line. The meanings of these symbols will be shown in the LEGEND. Specific features that do appear in the legend will be labeled on the map itself.

The spatial relationship between the features on a map is indicated both by their position on the page and by the SCALE, which shows the relationship between distance on the map and distance in real life. The scale will be a short line marked with a specific measurement like 100 kilometers or 10 miles. This measurement provides a conversion factor to find the real-life distance between features on the map. For example, if the scale line is 1 inch long and corresponds to 50 miles in real life, then 2 inches on the map equals 100 miles in real life, and so on.

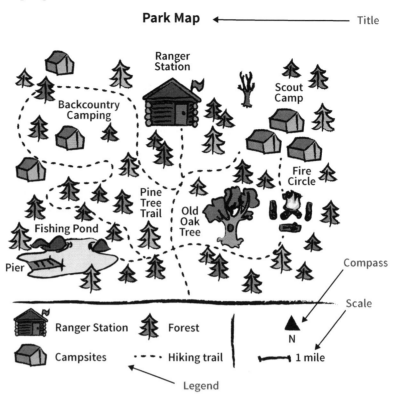

Figure 2.1. Map

Maps will also include a COMPASS, which shows the four cardinal directions: north, south, east, and west. Traditionally, maps are oriented with the top of the page being north and the right side of the page being east, although this is not an absolute.

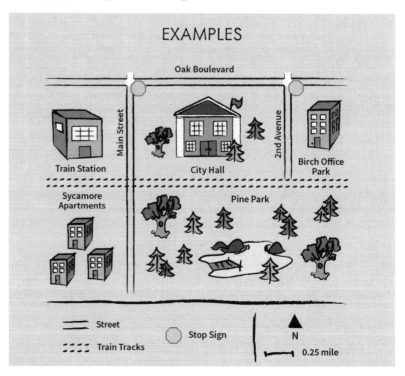

Graphs and Charts

GRAPHS and CHARTS are visual representations of data. These figures include line graphs, bar graphs, pie charts, scatter plots, and histograms. These figures have a number of key features that you will need to identify. Graphs and charts will always have a TITLE that provides a brief description of the data being described. The title will often include information that is vital for understanding the graph. For example, the title *Graduating Students in the Class of 2016* tells the reader that the data set to follow includes students who graduated in 2016. The graph may also include a SUBTITLE that provides more detailed information.

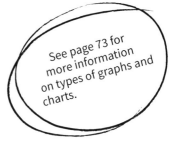

See page 73 for more information on types of graphs and charts.

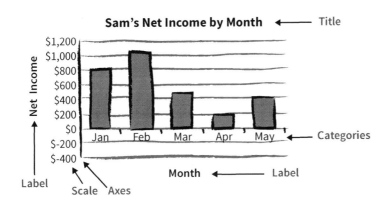

Figure 2.2. Sam's Income

Graphs also include horizontal and vertical AXES with LABELS describing the data being charted on each axis. Both labels should show the units of the data being displayed on that axis. Axes showing countable data, such as money or the number of students, will include a numeric SCALE that allows the reader to determine the value of each point or bar on the graph. Axes that show categorical data, such as time or location, will include text with the name for each category.

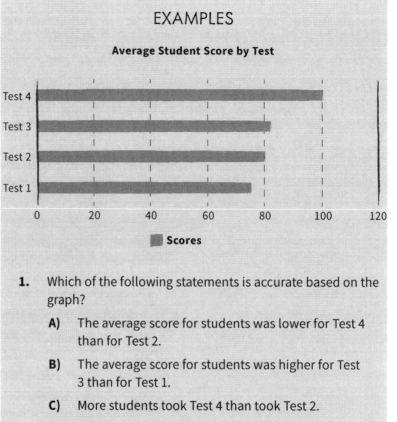

EXAMPLES

Average Student Score by Test

1. Which of the following statements is accurate based on the graph?

   A) The average score for students was lower for Test 4 than for Test 2.

   B) The average score for students was higher for Test 3 than for Test 1.

   C) More students took Test 4 than took Test 2.

   D) Fewer students took Test 3 than took Test 1.

   B) is correct. The title of the graph states that the bars show the average student score, not the number of students who took the test. The bar length shows that the average student score was higher for Test 3 than for Test 1.

2. Which of the following features on a graph will show the units of the data being displayed?

   A) scale

   B) title

   C) axis label

   D) subtitle

   C) is correct. The axis label will show the units for the data shown on that axis.

Other Informational Figures

The TEAS Reading test will include questions about an assortment of other information figures, including flowcharts, diagrams, and print media like brochures and flyers. There's no simple set of rules for handling these questions, but many of the same strategies that are used for other figures and for text passages are applicable.

Always start with the title of a figure—it will provide information that is likely crucial to understanding the figure. An anatomical diagram might have a title such as *Lobes of the Brain* that tells the viewer that the diagram will likely show the names and locations of the brain's lobes. Similarly, a flyer for a local garage sale might have a title like *Biggest Garage Sale in the Neighborhood* that tells the viewer exactly what the flyer is promoting.

Also make sure to examine any labels, legends, or scales provided with the figure. Anatomical diagrams, for example, will likely include labels for specific anatomical features, and a flowchart will have arrows indicating an ordered sequence. These labels can be read just like they would be on a map or graph.

Many of the strategies needed to interpret traditional reading passages can also be used for graphic representations of information, particularly those that may be text heavy. When looking at a flyer or advertisement, it will help to identify:

- the purpose of the author
- the intended audience
- rhetorical strategies designed to influence the viewer

A flyer for a local bake sale, for example, may be designed to appeal to the viewer's emotions by including pictures of local school children. Similarly, a computer advertisement meant to appeal to corporate buyers would probably use more formal language than one aimed at teenagers.

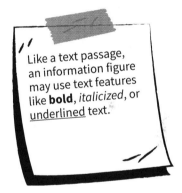

Most figures on the TEAS Reading will not require any outside knowledge to use. However, some questions may be easier if you have a basic understanding of common tools. For example, you may be asked to interpret the display for a blood pressure monitor or read a scale.

Like a text passage, an information figure may use text features like **bold**, *italicized*, or underlined text.

GO ON

EXAMPLES

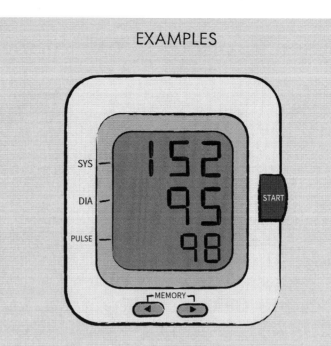

1. The device in the illustration above is used to measure which of the following?

   A) bone density

   B) tidal volume

   C) blood sugar

   D) blood pressure

   D) is correct. The illustration shows the display from a blood pressure monitor; the display gives systolic pressure, diastolic pressure, and heart rate.

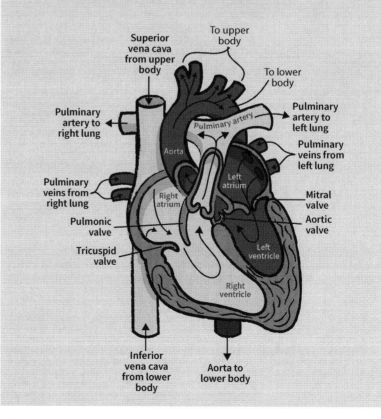

2. According to the figure, which of the following separates the right atrium from the right ventricle?

   A) mitral valve

   B) tricuspid valve

   C) aortic valve

   D) pulmonic valve

   B) is correct. The diagram shows that the tricuspid valve is located between the right atrium and the right ventricle.

Following Directions

DIRECTIONS provide step-by-step instructions for completing a particular task; these appear in all aspects of life, from instructions on microwave dinners to best practices for sterile technique. On the TEAS, directions may appear as simple lists, although they are often accompanied by shapes or figures to be manipulated as part of the directions. For example, a question may present a series of shapes, each of which may be rotated, moved, or deleted as designated by the directions.

Following directions requires the ability to identify the initial conditions, understand sequences, and analyze relationships among steps. First, identify the initial conditions laid out by the problem. This might be a spatial relationship between figures or a certain number of items (e.g., three red marbles and two green marbles).

Next, look for markers that indicate sequence. That may be as simple as identifying numbered steps, or the problem might require a closer reading. Certain words provide clues to the sequence of steps. Transition words like *first*, *next*, *then*, and *finally* indicate the order of tasks to be carried out. Once the order of steps has been identified, they can be carried out in that order.

When working through directions, pay special attention to the relationships between the steps. The action carried out in step 1 will likely affect the action in step 2, so make sure that each step is completed correctly before moving on. These questions are a test of the reader's attention to detail.

When working through a set of directions, ALWAYS write down the result of each step. This will help you avoid making simple mistakes and will also help you check your work if you find an error.

GO ON

EXAMPLES

Directions:

1. Imagine three apples, two oranges, and two limes in a fruit bowl.

2. Remove one apple.

3. Add two oranges.

4. Add one lime.

5. Add three apples.

6. Remove one orange.

1. Which of the following is the number of each fruit now in the bowl?

   A) 4 apples, 2 oranges, 3 limes

   B) 4 apples, 4 oranges, 2 limes

   C) 5 apples, 3 oranges, 3 limes

   D) 5 apples, 4 oranges, 2 limes

   C) is correct. Following the directions step by step gives the following number of fruit:

   1. **3 apples, 2 oranges, 2 limes**

   2. **2 apples, 2 oranges, 2 limes**

   3. **2 apples, 4 oranges, 2 limes**

   4. **2 apples, 4 oranges, 3 limes**

   5. **5 apples, 4 oranges, 3 limes**

   6. **5 apples, 3 oranges, 3 limes**

2. Start with the figure below. Follow the directions.

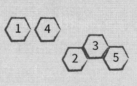

   1. Remove block 3.

   2. Place block 4 where block 3 used to be.

   3. Swap blocks 1 and 2.

   4. Move block 5 up one spot.

   5. Place block 3 where block 5 used to be.

Which of the following is the resulting arrangement of the blocks?

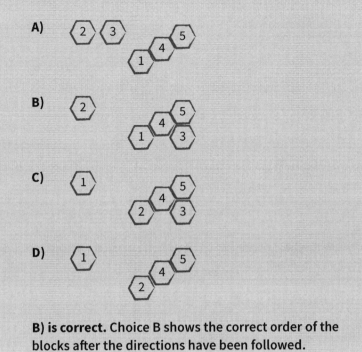

A)

B)

C)

D)

B) is correct. Choice B shows the correct order of the blocks after the directions have been followed.

PART II: MATHEMATICS

three

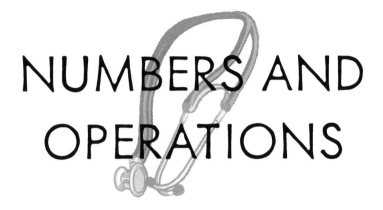

NUMBERS AND OPERATIONS

Types of Numbers

Numbers are placed in categories based on their properties.

- A **NATURAL NUMBER** is greater than zero and has no decimal or fraction attached. These are also sometimes called counting numbers. {1, 2, 3, 4, ...}

- **WHOLE NUMBERS** are natural numbers and the number zero. {0, 1, 2, 3, 4, ...}

- **INTEGERS** include positive and negative natural numbers and zero. {. . ., -4, -3, -2, -1, 0, 1, 2, 3, 4, ...}

- A **RATIONAL NUMBER** can be represented as a fraction. Any decimal part must terminate, or resolve into a repeating pattern. Examples include -12, $-\frac{4}{5}$, 0.36, $7.\overline{7}$, $26\frac{1}{2}$, etc.

- An **IRRATIONAL NUMBER** cannot be represented as a fraction. An irrational decimal number never ends and never resolves into a repeating pattern. Examples include $-\sqrt{7}$, Π, and 0.34567989135 ...

- A **REAL NUMBER** is a number that can be represented by a point on a number line. Real numbers include all the rational and irrational numbers.

If a real number is a natural number (e.g. 50), then it is also an integer, a whole number, and a rational number. .

Every whole number (except 1) is either a prime number or a composite number. A **PRIME NUMBER** is a natural number greater than 1 which can only be divided evenly by 1 and itself. For example 7 is a prime number because it can only be divided by the numbers 1 and 7.

On the other hand, a **COMPOSITE NUMBER** is a natural number greater than 1 which can be evenly divided by at least one other

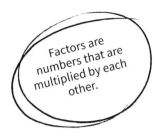

Factors are numbers that are multiplied by each other.

number besides 1 and itself. For example, 6 is a composite number because it can be divided by 1, 2, 3, and 6.

Composite numbers can be broken down into prime numbers using factor trees. For example, the number 54 is 2 × 27, and 27 is 3 × 9, and 9 is 3 × 3, as shown in the figure below.

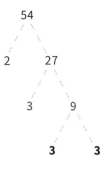

Figure 3.1. Factor Tree

Once the number has been broken down into its simplest form, the composite number can be expressed using exponents. An **EXPONENT** shows how many times a number should be multiplied by itself. In the factor tree, the number 54 can be written as $2 \times 3 \times 3 \times 3$ or 2×3^3.

EXAMPLES

Classify the following numbers as natural, whole, integer, rational, or irrational. (The numbers may have more than one classification.)

1. 72

   natural, whole, integer, and rational (72 can be written as the fraction $\frac{72}{1}$)

2. $-\frac{2}{3}$

   rational (the number is a fraction)

3. $\sqrt{5}$

   irrational (the number cannot be written as a fraction, and written as a decimal it is approximately 2.2360679... Notice this decimal does not terminate, nor does it have a repeating pattern.)

Scientific Notation

SCIENTIFIC NOTATION is a method of representing very large and small numbers in the form $a \times 10^n$ where a is a value between 1 and 10, and n is a nonzero integer. For example, the number 927,000,000 is written in scientific notation as 9.27×10^8. Multiplying 9.27 by 10 eight times gives 927,000,000. When performing operations with scientific notation, the final answer should be in the form $a \times 10^n$.

Table 3.1. Place Value

1,000,000	100,000	10,000	1,000	100	1	•	1/10	1/100
10^6	10^5	10^4	10^3	10^2	10^1		10^{-1}	10^{-2}
Millions	Hundred Thousands	Ten Thousands	Thousands	Hundreds	Tens	Decimal	Tenths	Hundreths

When adding and subtracting numbers in scientific notation, the power of 10 must be the same for all numbers. This results in like terms in which the *a* terms are added or subtracted and the 10^n remains unchanged. When multiplying numbers in scientific notation, multiply the *a* factors and add the exponents. For division, divide the *a* factors and subtract the exponents.

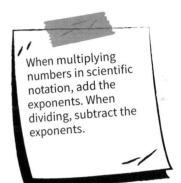

When multiplying numbers in scientific notation, add the exponents. When dividing, subtract the exponents.

EXAMPLES

1. Simplify: $(3.8 \times 10^3) + (4.7 \times 10^2)$

   In order to add, the exponents of 10 must be the same. Change the first number so the power of 10 is 2:

   $38 \times 10^3 = 3.8 \times 10 \times 10^2 = 38 \times 10^2$

   Add the *a* terms together and write the number in proper scientific notation:

   $3.8 \times 10^2 + 4.7 \times 10^2 = 42.7 \times 10^2 = 4.27 \times 10^3$

2. Simplify: $(8.1 \times 10^{-5})(1.4 \times 10^7)$

   Multiply the *a* factors and add the exponents on the base of 10:

   $(8.1 \times 1.4)(10^{-5} \times 10^7) = 11.34 \times 10^2$

   Write the number in proper scientific notation: (Place the decimal so that the first number is between 1 and 10 and adjust the exponent accordingly.)

   $11.34 \times 10^2 = 1.134 \times 10^3$

Positive and Negative Numbers

POSITIVE NUMBERS are greater than zero, and NEGATIVE NUMBERS are less than zero. Both positive and negative numbers can be shown on a NUMBER LINE.

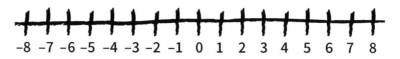

Figure 3.2. Number Line

Positive and negative numbers can be added, subtracted, multiplied, and divided. The sign of the resulting number is governed by a specific set of rules shown in the table below.

Table 1.2. Operations with Positive and Negative Numbers

ADDING REAL NUMBERS

Positve + Positive = Positive	$7 + 8 = 15$
Negative + Negative = Negative	$-7 + (-8) = -15$
Negative + Positive = OR Positive + Negative = Keep the sign of the number with the larger absolute value and subtract the absolute values of the numbers	$-7 + 8 = 1$ $7 + (-8) = -1$

SUBTRACTING REAL NUMBERS

Change the subtraction to addition, change the sign of the second number, and use addition rules.

Negative – Positive = Negative	$-7 - 8 = -7 + (-8) = -15$
Positive – Negative = Positive	$7 - (-8) = 7 + 8 = 15$
Negative – Negative = Keep the sign of the number with the larger absolute value and subtract the absolute values of the numbers	$-7 - (-8) = -7 + 8 = 1$ $-8 - (-7) = -8 + 7 = -1$

MULTIPLYING REAL NUMBERS

Positive × Positive = Positive	$8 \times 4 = 32$
Negative × Negative = Positive	$-8 \times (-4) = 32$
Positive × Negative OR Negative × Positive = Negative	$8 \times (-4) = -32$ $-8 \times 4 = -32$

DIVIDING REAL NUMBERS

Positive ÷ Positive = Positive	$8 \div 4 = 2$
Negative ÷ Negative = Positive	$-8 \div (-4) = 2$
Positive ÷ Negative OR Negative ÷ Positive = Negative	$8 \div (-4) = -2$ $-8 \div 4 = -2$

EXAMPLES

Add or subtract the following real numbers:

1. $-18 + 12$

    Since $|-18| > |12|$, the answer is negative. $|-18| - |12| = 6$. So the answer is -6.

2. −3.64 + (−2.18)

Adding two negative numbers results in a negative number. Add the values: −5.82

3. 9.37 − 4.25

5.12

4. 86 − (−20)

Change the subtraction to addition, change the sign of the second number, then add:
8 − (−20) = 86 + (+20) = 106

Multiply or divide the following real numbers:

5. $\frac{10}{3}\left(-\frac{9}{5}\right)$

Multiply the numerators, multiply the denominators, then simplify: $\frac{-90}{15} = -6$

6. $\frac{-64}{-10}$

A negative divided by a negative is a positive number:
6.4

7. (2.2)(3.3)

The parentheses indicate multiplication: 7.26

8. −52 ÷ 13

−4

Order of Operations

When solving a multi-step equation, the **ORDER OF OPERATIONS** must be used to get the correct answer. Generally speaking, the problem should be worked in the following order: 1) parenthesis and brackets; 2) exponents and square roots; 3) multiplication and division; 4) addition and subtraction. The acronym PEMDAS can be used to remember the order of operations.

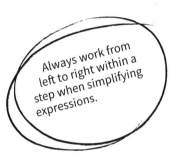

Always work from left to right within a step when simplifying expressions.

Please **E**xcuse (**M**y **D**ear) (**A**unt **S**ally)

1. **P** — Parenthesis: Calculate expressions inside parenthesis, brackets, braces, etc.
2. **E** — Exponents: Calculate exponents and square roots.
3. **M** — Multiply and **D** — Divide: Calculate any remaining multiplication and division in order from left to right.
4. **A** — Add and **S** — Subtract: Calculate any remaining addition and subtraction in order from left to right.

The steps "Multiply-Divide" and "Addition-Subtraction" go in order from left to right. In other words, divide before multiplying if the division problem is on the left.

For example, the expression $(3^2 - 2)^2 + (4)5^3$ is simplified using the following steps:

1. Parentheses: Because the parentheses in this problem contain two operations (exponents and subtraction) use the order of operations within the parenthesis. Exponents come before subtraction.
   $(3^2 - 2)^2 + (4)5^3 = (9 - 2)^2 + (4)5^3 = (7)^2 + (4)5^3$

2. Exponents:
   $(7)^2 + (4)5^3 = 49 + (4)125$

3. Multiplication and division:
   $49 + (4)125 = 49 + 500$

4. Addition and subtraction:
   $49 + 500 = 549$

EXAMPLES

1. Simplify: $2(21 - 14) + 6 \div (-2) \times 3 - 10$

   Calculate the expressions inside the parenthesis:

   $2(21 - 14) + 6 \div (-2) \times 3 - 10 =$

   $2(7) + 6 \div (-2) \times 3 - 10$

   There are no exponents or radicals, so perform multiplication and division from left to right:

   $2(7) + 6 \div (-2) \times 3 - 10 =$

   $14 + 6 \div (-2) \times 3 - 10 =$

   $14 + (-3) \times 3 - 10 =$

   $14 + (-9) - 10$

   Lastly, perform addition and subtraction from left to right:

   $14 + (-9) - 10 =$

   $5 - 10 =$

   -5

2. Simplify: $-3^2 + 4(5) + (5 - 6)^2 - 8$

   Calculate the expressions inside the parenthesis:

   $-(3)^2 + 4(5) + (5 - 6)^2 - 8 =$

   $-(3)^2 + 4(5) + (-1)^2 - 8$

   Simplify exponents and radicals:

   $-(3)^2 + 4(5) + (-1)^2 - 8 =$

   $-9 + 4(5) + 1 - 8$

   Note that $-(3)^2 = -1(3)^2 = -9$ but $(-1)^2 = (-1)(-1) = 1$

   Perform multiplication and division from left to right:

   $-9 + 4(5) + 1 - 8 =$

   $-9 + 20 + 1 - 8$

Lastly, perform addition and subtraction from left to right:

$-9 + 20 + 1 - 8 =$

$11 + 1 - 8 =$

$12 - 8 =$

4

3. Simplify: $\dfrac{(7 - 9)^3 + 8(10 - 12)}{4^2 - 5^2}$

Simplify the top and bottom expressions separately using the same steps described above:

$\dfrac{(-2)^3 + 8(-2)}{4^2 - 5^2} =$

$\dfrac{(-2)^3 + (-16)}{4^2 - 5^2} =$

$\dfrac{-8 + (-16)}{16 - 25} =$

$\dfrac{-24}{-9} =$

$\dfrac{8}{3}$

Decimals and Fractions

Decimals

A **DECIMAL** is a number that contains a decimal point. The place value for a decimal includes **TENTHS** (one place after the decimal), **HUNDREDTHS** (two places after the decimal), and **THOUSANDTHS** (three places after the decimal), etc.

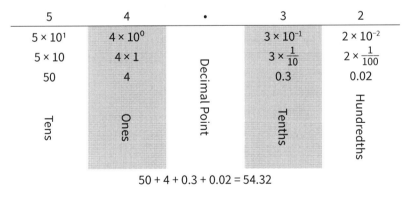

$$50 + 4 + 0.3 + 0.02 = 54.32$$

Figure 3.3. Decimals and Place Value

Decimals can be added, subtracted, multiplied, and divided:

To add or subtract decimals, line up the decimal point and perform the operation, keeping the decimal point in the same place in the answer.

$$
\begin{array}{r}
12.35 \\
+\ 3.63 \\
\hline
= 15.98
\end{array}
$$

To multiply decimals, first multiply the numbers without the decimal points. Then, add the number of decimal places to the right of the decimal point in the original numbers and place the decimal point in the answer so that there are that many places to the right of the decimal.

$$12.35 \times 3.63 =$$

$$1235 \times 363 = 448305 \rightarrow 44.8305$$

When dividing decimals move the decimal point to the right in order to make the divisor a whole number and move the decimal the same number places in the dividend. Divide the numbers without regard to the decimal. Then, place the decimal point of the quotient directly above the decimal point of the dividend.

$$\frac{12.35}{3.63} = \frac{1235}{363} =$$

$$\begin{array}{r} 3.40 \\ 363 \overline{\smash{\big)}\ 1235.00} \end{array}$$

Sidebar note:

> If you're unsure which way to move the decimal after multiplying, remember that changing the decimal should always make the final answer smaller.

EXAMPLES

1. Simplify: 24.38 + 16.51 − 29.87

    Apply the order of operations left to right:

    24.38 + 16.51 = 40.89

    40.89 − 29.87 =

    11.02

2. Simplify: (10.4)(18.2)

    Multiply the numbers ignoring the decimals:

    104 × 182 = 18,928

    The original problem includes two decimal places (10.4 has one place after the decimal point and 18.2 has one place after the decimal point), so place the decimal point in the answer so that there are two places after the decimal point. Estimating is a good way to check the answer (10.4 ≈ 10, 18.2 ≈ 18, *and* 10 × 18 = 180)

    18,928 → 189.28

3. Simplify: 80 ÷ 2.5

    The divisor is 2.5. Move the decimal one place to the right (multiply 2.5 by 10) so that the divisor is a whole number. Since the decimal point of the divisor was moved one place to the right, the decimal point in the dividend must be moved one place right (multiplying it by 10 as well).

    80 → 800 and 2.5 → 25

    Divide normally: 800 ÷ 25 = **32**

Fractions

A fraction is a number that can be written in the form $\frac{a}{b}$ where b is not equal to zero. The a part of the fraction is the numerator (top number) and b part of the fraction is the denominator (bottom number).

If the denominator of a fraction is greater than the numerator, the value of the fraction is less than 1 and it is called a proper fraction (e.g., $\frac{3}{5}$ is a proper fraction).

In an **IMPROPER FRACTION**, the denominator is less than the numerator and the value of the fraction is greater than one (e.g., $\frac{8}{3}$ is an improper fraction). An improper fraction can be written as a mixed number. A **MIXED NUMBER** has a whole number part and a proper fraction part. Improper fractions can be converted to mixed numbers by dividing the numerator by the denominator, which gives the whole number part, and the remainder becomes the numerator of the proper fraction part (for example: improper fraction $\frac{25}{9}$ is equal to mixed number $2\frac{7}{9}$ because 9 divides into 25 two times, with a remainder of 7).

Conversely, mixed numbers can be converted to improper fractions. To do so, determine the numerator of the improper fraction by multiplying the denominator by the whole number, then adding the numerator. The final number is written as the (now larger) numerator over the original denominator.

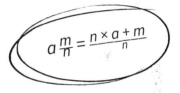

$$a\frac{m}{n} = \frac{n \times a + m}{n}$$

Fractions with the same denominator can be added or subtracted by simply adding or subtracting the numerators; the denominator will remain unchanged. If the fractions to be added or subtracted do not have a common denominator, the least common multiple of the denominators must be found. The quickest way to find a common denominator of a set of values is simply to multiply all the values together. The result might not be the least common denominator, but it will get the job done. Any common denominator can be used to add or subtract fractions, but using the least common denominator means the problem will not have to be simplified later.

In the operation $\frac{2}{3} - \frac{1}{2}$, the common denominator will be a multiple of both 3 and 2. Multiples are found by multiplying the denominator by whole numbers until a common multiple is found:

- multiples of 3 are **3** (3 × 1), **6** (3 × 2), **9** (3 × 3) …
- multiples of 2 are **2** (2 × 1), **4** (2 × 2), **6** (2 × 3) …

Since 6 is the smallest multiple of both 3 and 2, it is the least common multiple and can be used as the common denominator. Both the numerator and denominator of each fraction should be multiplied by the appropriate whole number:

$$\frac{2}{3}\left(\frac{2}{2}\right) - \frac{1}{2}\left(\frac{3}{3}\right) = \frac{4}{6} - \frac{3}{6} = \frac{1}{6}.$$

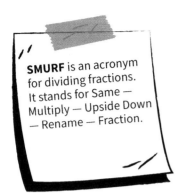

When multiplying fractions, simply multiply each numerator together and each denominator together. To divide two fractions, invert the second fraction (swap the numerator and denominator) then multiply normally. If there are any mixed numbers when multiplying or dividing, they should first be changed to improper fractions. Note that multiplying fractions creates a value smaller than either original value.

- $\frac{5}{6} \times \frac{2}{3} = \frac{10}{18} = \frac{5}{9}$
- $\frac{5}{6} \div \frac{2}{3} = \frac{5}{6} \times \frac{3}{2} = \frac{15}{12} = \frac{5}{4}$

EXAMPLES

1. Simplify: $2\frac{3}{5} + 3\frac{1}{4} - 1\frac{1}{2}$

   The first step is to change each fraction so it has a denominator of 20, which is the LCD of 5, 4, and 2:

   $2\frac{3}{5} + 3\frac{1}{4} - 1\frac{1}{2} = 2\frac{12}{20} + 3\frac{5}{20} - 1\frac{10}{20}$

   Next, add and subtract the whole numbers together and the fractions together:

   $2 + 3 - 1 = 4$

   $\frac{12}{20} + \frac{5}{20} - \frac{10}{20} = \frac{7}{20}$

   Lastly, combine to get the final answer (a mixed number):

   $4\frac{7}{20}$

2. Simplify: $\frac{7}{8}\left(3\frac{1}{3}\right)$

   Change the mixed number to an improper fraction:

   $3\frac{1}{3} = \frac{10}{3}$

   Multiply the numerators together and the denominators together, and then reduce the fraction:

   $\frac{7}{8}\left(\frac{10}{3}\right) = \frac{7 \times 10}{8 \times 3} = \frac{70}{24} = \frac{35}{12} =$

   $2\frac{11}{12}$

3. Simplify: $4\frac{1}{2} \div \frac{2}{3}$

   Change the mixed number to an improper fraction. Then, multiply the first fraction by the reciprocal of the second fraction and simplify:

   $\frac{9}{2} \div \frac{2}{3} = \frac{9}{2} \times \frac{3}{2} = \frac{27}{4} =$

   $6\frac{3}{4}$

Converting Between Fractions and Decimals

A fraction is converted to a decimal by using long division until there is no remainder or a pattern of repeating numbers occurs.

$$\frac{1}{2} = 1 \div 2 = 0.5$$

To convert a decimal to a fraction, place the numbers to the right of the decimal over the appropriate base-10 power and simplify the fraction.

$$0.375 = \frac{375}{1000} = \frac{3}{8}$$

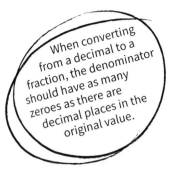

When converting from a decimal to a fraction, the denominator should have as many zeroes as there are decimal places in the original value.

EXAMPLES

1. Write the fraction $\frac{7}{8}$ as a decimal.

    Divide the denominator into the numerator using long division:

    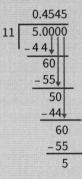

    ```
         0.875
      8 │ 7.000
        −64
          60
         −56
          60
         −56
           40
          −40
            0
    ```

2. Write the fraction $\frac{5}{11}$ as a decimal.

    Dividing using long division yields a repeating decimal:

    ```
          0.4545
      11 │ 5.0000
         −44
           60
          −55
            50
           −44
             60
            −55
              5
    ```

3. Write the decimal 0.125 as a fraction.

    Create a fraction with 0.125 as the numerator and 1 as the denominator:

    $$0.125 = \frac{0.125}{1}$$

    Multiply by 1 in the form $\frac{10}{10}$ three times (one for each numeral after the decimal), and then simplify:

    $$\frac{0.125}{1} \times \frac{10}{10} \times \frac{10}{10} \times \frac{10}{10} = \frac{125}{1000} = \frac{1}{8}$$

    Alternately, recognize that 0.125 is read as "one hundred twenty-five thousandths" and can therefore be written in fraction form as $\frac{125}{1000}$.

GO ON

Rounding and Estimation

ROUNDING is a way of simplifying a complicated number. The result of rounding will be a less precise value that is easier to write or perform operations on. Rounding is performed to a specific place value, such as the thousands or tenths place.

The rules for rounding are as follows:

1. Underline the place value being rounded to.
2. Locate the digit one place value to the right of the underlined value. If this value is less than 5, keep the underlined value and replace all digits to the right of the underlined value with zero. If the value to the right of the underlined digit is more than 5, increase the underlined digit by one and replace all digits to the right of it with zero.

ESTIMATION is when numbers are rounded and then an operation is performed. This process can be used when working with large numbers to find a close, but not exact, answer.

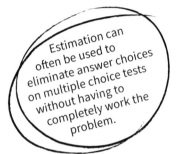
Estimation can often be used to eliminate answer choices on multiple choice tests without having to completely work the problem.

EXAMPLES

1. Round the number 138,472 to the nearest thousands.

The 8 is in the thousands place, and the number to its right is a 4. Because 4 is less than 5, the 8 remains and all numbers to the right become zero:

138,472 ≈ 138,000

2. The populations of five local towns are 12,341, 8,975, 9,431, 10,521, and 11,427. Estimate the population to the nearest 1,000 people.

Round each value to the thousands place and add:

12,341 ≈ 12,000

8,975 ≈ 9,000

9,431 ≈ 9,000

10,521 ≈ 11,000

11,427 ≈ 11,000

12,000 + 9,000 + 9,000 + 11,000 + 11,000 =

52,000

Ratios

A RATIO is a comparison of two numbers and can be represented as $\frac{a}{b} (b \neq 0)$, $a:b$, or a to b. The two numbers represent a constant relationship, not a specific value: for every a number of items in the first group, there will be b number of items in the second. For example, if the ratio of blue to red candies in a bag is 3:5, the bag will contain 3 blue candies for every 5 red candies. So, the bag might contain 3 blue candies and 5 red candies, or it might contain 30 blue candies and 50 red candies, or 36 blue candies and 60 red candies. All of these values are representative of the ratio 3:5 (which is the ratio in its lowest, or simplest, terms).

To find the "whole" when working with ratios, simply add the values in the ratio. For example, if the ratio of boys to girls in a class is 2:3, the "whole" is five: 2 out of every 5 students are boys, and 3 out of every 5 students are girls.

EXAMPLES

1. There are 10 boys and 12 girls in a first grade class. What is the ratio of boys to the total number of students? What is the ratio of girls to boys?

There are 22 total students in the class. The ratio can be written as $\frac{10}{22}$, and reduced to $\frac{5}{11}$. The ratio of girls to boys is 12:10 or 6:5.

2. A family spends $600 a month on rent, $400 on utilities, $750 on groceries, and $550 on miscellaneous expenses. What is the ratio of the family's rent to their total expenses?

The family's total expenses for the month add up to $2,300. The ratio for the rent to total amount of expenses can be written as $\frac{600}{2300}$ and reduced to $\frac{6}{23}$.

Proportions

A **PROPORTION** is an equation which states that two ratios are equal. Proportions are given in the form $\frac{a}{b} = \frac{c}{d}$, where the a and d terms are the extremes and the b and c terms are the means. A proportion is solved using **CROSS-MULTIPLICATION** to create an equation with no fractional components: $\frac{a}{b} = \frac{c}{d} \rightarrow ad = bc$

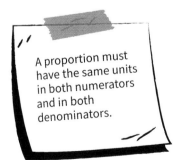

A proportion must have the same units in both numerators and in both denominators.

EXAMPLES

1. Solve the proportion for x: $\frac{3x-5}{2} = \frac{x-8}{3}$.

Start by cross multiplying:

$\frac{3x-5}{2} = \frac{x-8}{3} \rightarrow 3(3x-5) = 2(x-8)$

Then, solve the equation for x:

$9x - 15 = 2x - 16$

$7x - 15 = -16$

$7x = -1$

$x = -\frac{1}{7}$

2. A map is drawn such that 2.5 inches on the map equates to an actual distance of 40 miles. If the distance measured on the map between two cities is 17.25 inches, what is the actual distance between them in miles?

Write a proportion where x equals the actual distance and each ratio is written as inches : miles.

$$\frac{2.5}{40} = \frac{17.25}{x}$$

Then, cross-multiply and divide to solve for x:

$2.5x = 690$

$x = 276$

The two cities are 276 miles apart.

3. A factory knows that every 4 out of 1,000 parts made will be defective. If in a month there are 125,000 parts made, how many of these parts will be defective?

Write a proportion in which x is the number of defective parts made and both ratios are written as defective : total.

$$\frac{4}{1000} = \frac{x}{125,000}$$

Then, cross-multiply and divide to solve for x:

$1000x = 500,000$

$x = 500$

There are 500 defective parts for the month.

Percentages

A PERCENT (or percentage) means per hundred and is expressed with a percent symbol (%). For example, 54% means 54 out of every 100. A percent can be converted to a decimal by removing the % symbol and moving the decimal point two places to the left, while a decimal can be converted to a percent by moving the decimal point two places to the right and attaching the % sign.

A percent can be converted to a fraction by writing the percent as a fraction with 100 as the denominator and reducing. A fraction can be converted to a percent by performing the indicated division, multiplying the result by 100 and attaching the % sign.

The equation for finding percentages has three variables: the part, the whole, and the percent (which is expressed in the equation as a decimal). The equation, as shown below, can be rearranged to solve for any of these variables.

$$part = whole \times percent$$
$$percent = \frac{part}{whole}$$
$$whole = \frac{part}{percent}$$

This set of equations can be used to solve percent word problems. All that is needed is to identify the part, whole, and/or percent, then to plug those values into the appropriate equation and solve.

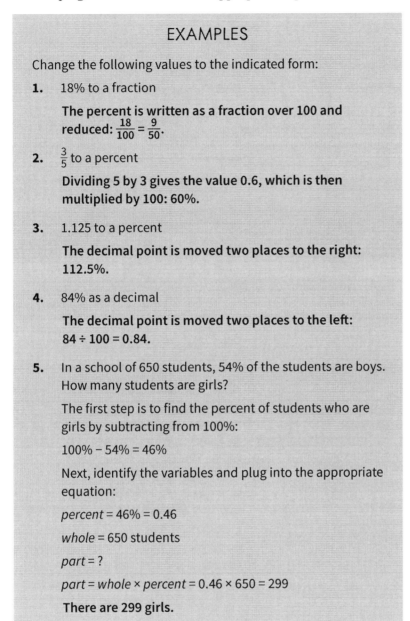

EXAMPLES

Change the following values to the indicated form:

1. 18% to a fraction

    The percent is written as a fraction over 100 and reduced: $\frac{18}{100} = \frac{9}{50}$.

2. $\frac{3}{5}$ to a percent

    Dividing 5 by 3 gives the value 0.6, which is then multiplied by 100: 60%.

3. 1.125 to a percent

    The decimal point is moved two places to the right: 112.5%.

4. 84% as a decimal

    The decimal point is moved two places to the left: $84 \div 100 = 0.84$.

5. In a school of 650 students, 54% of the students are boys. How many students are girls?

    The first step is to find the percent of students who are girls by subtracting from 100%:

    100% − 54% = 46%

    Next, identify the variables and plug into the appropriate equation:

    $percent = 46\% = 0.46$

    $whole = 650$ students

    $part = ?$

    $part = whole \times percent = 0.46 \times 650 = 299$

    There are 299 girls.

Percent Change

Percent change problems involve a change from an original amount. Often percent change problems appear as word problems that include discounts, growth, or markups. In order to solve percent change problems, it is necessary to identify the percent change (as a decimal), the amount of change, and the original amount. (Keep in mind that one of these will be the value being solved for.) These values can then be plugged into the equations below:

$$amount\ of\ change = original\ amount \times percent\ change$$
$$percent\ change = \frac{amount\ of\ change}{original\ amount}$$

$$original\ amount = \frac{amount\ of\ change}{percent\ change}$$

EXAMPLES

1. A Smart HDTV that originally cost $1,500 is on sale for 45% off. What is the sale price for the item?

   The first step is to identify the necessary values. These can then be plugged into the appropriate equation:

   original amount = 1,500

   percent change = 45% = 0.45

   amount of change = ?

   amount of change = *original amount* × *percent change* = 1,500 × 0.45 = 675

   To find the new price, subtract the amount of change from the original price:

   1,500 – 675 = 825

   The final price is $825.

2. A house was purchased in 2000 for $100,000 and sold in 2015 for $120,000. What was the percent growth in the value of the house from 2000 to 2015?

   Identify the necessary values and plug into the appropriate equation:

   original amount = 100,000

   amount of change = 120,000 – 100,000 = 20,000

   percent change = ?

   $percent\ change = \frac{amount\ of\ change}{original\ amount} = \frac{20,000}{100,000} = 0.20$

   To find the percent growth, multiply by 100:

   0.20 × 100 = 20%

Comparison of Rational Numbers

Rational numbers can be ordered from least to greatest (or greatest to least) by placing them in the order in which they fall on a number line. When comparing a set of fractions, it is often easiest to convert each value to a common denominator. Then, it is only necessary to compare the numerators of each fraction.

When working with numbers in multiple forms (for example, a group of fractions and decimals), convert the values so that the set contains only fractions or only decimals. When ordering negative numbers, remember that the negative numbers with the largest absolute values are furthest from 0 and are therefore the smallest numbers. (For example, –75 is smaller than –25.)

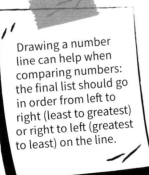

EXAMPLES

1. Order the following numbers from greatest to least:
   $-\frac{2}{3}, 1.2, 0, -2.1, \frac{5}{4}, -1, \frac{1}{8}$.

   Change each fraction to a decimal:

   $-\frac{2}{3} = -0.\overline{66}$

   $\frac{5}{4} = 1.25$

   $\frac{1}{8} = 0.125$

   Now place the decimals in order from greatest to least:

   $1.25, 1.2, 0.125, 0, -0.\overline{66}, -1, -2.1$

   Lastly, convert back to fractions if the problem requires it:

   $\frac{5}{4}, 1.2, \frac{1}{8}, 0, -\frac{2}{3}, -1, -2.1$

2. Order the following numbers from least to greatest:
   $\frac{1}{3}, -\frac{5}{6}, 1\frac{1}{8}, \frac{7}{12}, -\frac{3}{4}, -\frac{3}{2}$

   Convert each value using the least common denominator value of 24:

   $\frac{1}{3} = \frac{8}{24}$

   $-\frac{5}{6} = -\frac{20}{24}$

   $1\frac{1}{8} = \frac{9}{8} = \frac{27}{24}$

   $\frac{7}{12} = \frac{14}{24}$

   $-\frac{3}{4} = -\frac{18}{24}$

   $-\frac{3}{2} = -\frac{36}{24}$

   Next, put the fractions in order from least to greatest by comparing the numerators:

   $-\frac{36}{24}, -\frac{20}{24}, -\frac{18}{24}, \frac{8}{24}, \frac{14}{24}, \frac{27}{24}$

   Finally, put the fractions back in their original form if the problem requires it:

   $-\frac{3}{2}, -\frac{5}{6}, -\frac{3}{4}, \frac{1}{3}, \frac{7}{12}, 1\frac{1}{8}$

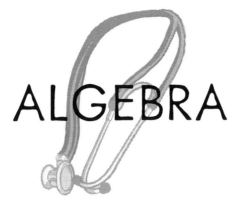

four

ALGEBRA

Algebraic Expressions

The foundation of algebra is the **VARIABLE**, an unknown number represented by a symbol (usually a letter such as x or a). Variables can be preceded by a **COEFFICIENT**, which is a constant (i.e., a real number) in front of the variable, such as $4x$ or $-2a$. An **ALGEBRAIC EXPRESSION** is any sum, difference, product, or quotient of variables and numbers (for example $3x^2$, $2x + 7y - 1$, and $\frac{5}{x}$ are algebraic expressions). **TERMS** are any quantities that are added or subtracted (for example the terms of the expression $x^2 - 3x + 5$ are x^2, $3x$, and 5). A **POLYNOMIAL EXPRESSION** is an algebraic expression where all the exponents on the variables are whole numbers. A polynomial with only two terms is known as a **BINOMIAL**, and one with three terms is a **TRINOMIAL**.

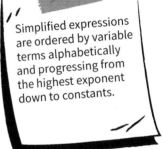

Simplified expressions are ordered by variable terms alphabetically and progressing from the highest exponent down to constants.

EXAMPLE

If $m = 4$, find the value of the following expression:

$5(m - 2)^3 + 3m^2 - \frac{m}{4} - 1$

First, plug the value 4 in for m in the expression:

Then, simplify using PEMDAS:

P: $5(2)^3 + 3(4)^2 - \frac{4}{4} - 1$

E: $5(8) + 3(16) - \frac{4}{4} - 1$

M/D at the same time, working left to right: $40 + 48 - 1 - 1$

A/S at the same time, working left to right: 86

The answer is 86.

Operations with Expressions

Adding and Subtracting

Expressions can be added or subtracted by simply adding and subtracting LIKE TERMS, which are terms with the same variable part (the variables must be the same, with the same exponents on each variable). For example, in the expressions $2x + 3xy - 2z$ and $6y + 2xy$, the like terms are $3xy$ and $2xy$. Adding the two expressions yields the new expression $2x + 5xy - 2z + 6y$. Note that the other terms did not change; they cannot combine because they have different variables.

EXAMPLE

If $a = 12x + 7xy - 9y$ and $b = 8x - 9xz + 7z$, what is $a + b$?

The only like terms in both expressions are $12x$ and $8x$, so these two terms will be added, and all other terms will remain the same:

$a + b = (12x + 8x) + 7xy - 9y - 9xz + 7z \rightarrow$

$20x + 7xy - 9y - 9xz + 7z$

Distributing and Factoring

Often, simplifying expressions requires distributing and factoring, which can be seen as two sides of the same coin. DISTRIBUTION multiplies each term in the first factor by each term in the second factor to clear off parentheses, while FACTORING reverses this process, taking a polynomial in standard form and writing it as a product of two or more factors.

When distributing a monomial through a polynomial, the expression outside the parentheses is multiplied by each term inside the parentheses. Remember, coefficients are multiplied and exponents are added, following the rules of exponents.

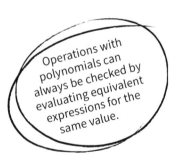

Operations with polynomials can always be checked by evaluating equivalent expressions for the same value.

The first step in factoring a polynomial is always to "undistribute" or factor out the greatest common factor (GCF) among the terms. The GCF is multiplied by, in parentheses, the expression that remains of each term when the GCF is divided out of each term. Factoring can be checked by multiplying the GCF factor through the parentheses again.

EXAMPLES

1. Expand the following expression: $5x(x^2 - 2c + 10)$

    The term outside the parenthesis must be distributed and multiplied to all three terms inside the parenthesis:

    $(5x)(x^2) = 5x^3$

$(5x)(-2c) = -10xc$

$(5x)(10) = 50x$

$5x(x^2 - 2c + 10) \rightarrow$

$5x^3 - 10xc + 50x$

2. Expand the following expression: $x(5 + z) - z(4x - z^2)$

   Start by distributing for each set of parentheses:

   $x(5 + z) - z(4x - z^2)$

   Notice that $-z$ is distributed and that $(-z)(-z^2) = +z^3$. **Failing to distribute the negative is a very common error.**

   $5x + xz - 4zx + z^3$

   Note that xz is a like term with zx (commutative property) and they can therefore be combined.

   Now combine like terms and place terms in the appropriate order (highest exponents first):

   $z^3 - 3xz + 5x$

Linear Equations

An EQUATION states that two expressions are equal to each other. Polynomial equations are categorized by the highest power of the variables they contain. For instance, the highest power of any exponent of a linear equation is 1, a quadratic equation has a variable raised to the second power, a cubic equation has a variable raised to the third power, and so on.

Solving Linear Equations

Solving an equation means finding the value(s) of the variable that make the equation true. To solve a linear equation, it is necessary to manipulate the terms so that the variable being solved for appears alone on exactly one side of the equal sign while everything else in the equation is on the other side.

The way to solve linear equations is to "undo" all the operations that connect numbers to the variable of interest. Follow these steps:

1. Eliminate fractions by multiplying each side by the least common multiple of any denominators.

2. Distribute to eliminate parentheses, braces, and brackets.

3. Combine like terms.

4. Use addition or subtraction to collect all terms containing the variable of interest to one side, and all terms not containing the variable to the other side.

5. Use multiplication or division to remove coefficients from the variable being solved for.

On multiple-choice tests, it is often easier to plug the possible values into the equation and determine which solution makes the equation true than to solve the equation.

Sometimes there are no numeric values in the equation, or there will be a mix of numerous variables and constants. The goal will be to solve the equation for one of the variables in terms of the other variables. In this case, the answer will be an expression involving numbers and letters instead of a numeric value.

EXAMPLES

1. Solve for x: $\dfrac{100(x+5)}{20} = 1$

   To cancel out the denominator, multiply both sides by 20:

   $20\dfrac{100(x+5)}{20} = 1 \times 20$

   $100(x+5) = 20$

   Next, distribute 100 through the parentheses:

   $100(x+5) = 20$

   $100x + 500 = 20$

   "Undo" the +500 by subtracting 500 from both sides of the equation to isolate the variable term:

   $100x = -480$

   Finally, "undo" the multiplication by 100: divide by 100 on both sides to solve for x:

   $x = \dfrac{-480}{100} = -4.8$

2. Solve for x: $2(x+2)^2 - 2x^2 + 10 = 20$

   First, simplify the left-hand side of the equation using order of operations and combining like terms.

   $2(x+2)^2 - 2x^2 + 10 = 20$

   Do the exponent first:

   $2(x+2)(x+2) - 2x^2 + 10 = 20$

   FOIL:

   $2(x^2 + 4x + 4) - 2x^2 + 10 = 20$

   Distribute the 2:

   $2x^2 + 8x + 8 - 2x^2 + 10 = 20$

   Combine like terms on the left-hand side:

   $8x + 18 = 42$

   Now, isolate the variable.

   "Undo" +18 by subtracting 18 from both sides: $8x + 18 = 20$

   $8x = 2$

   "Undo" multiplication by 8 by dividing both sides by 8:

   $x = \dfrac{2}{8}$ or $\dfrac{1}{4}$

3. Solve the equation for D: $\dfrac{A(3B+2D)}{2N} = 5M - 6$

   First, multiply both sides by $2N$ to clear the fraction, and distribute A through the parentheses:

$3AB + 2AD = 10MN - 12N$

Next, isolate the term with D by moving the $3AB$ term to the other side of the equation:

$2AD = 10MN - 12N - 3AB$

Finally, divide both sides by $2A$ to get D alone on the left hand side:

$D = \dfrac{10MN - 12N - 3AB}{2A}$

Graphs of Linear Equations

The most common way to write a linear equation is SLOPE-INTERCEPT FORM:

$$y = mx + b$$

In this equation, m is the SLOPE, which describes how steep the line is, and b is the Y-INTERCEPT. Slope is often described as "rise over run" because it is calculated as the difference in y-values (rise) over the difference in x-values (run). The slope of the line is also the RATE OF CHANGE of the dependent variable y with respect to the independent variable x. The y-intercept is the point where the line crosses the y-axis, or where x equals zero.

To graph a linear equation, identify the y-intercept and place that point on the y-axis. If the slope is not written as a fraction, make it a fraction by writing it over 1 $\left(\frac{m}{1}\right)$. Then use the slope to count up (or down if negative) the "rise" part of the slope and over the "run" part of the slope to find a second point. These points can then be connected to draw the line. To find the equation of a line, identify the y-intercept, if possible, on the graph and use two easily identifiable points to find the slope. If the y-intercept is not easily identified, identify the slope by choosing easily identifiable points, then choose one point on the graph, plug the point and the slope values into the equation, and solve for the missing value b.

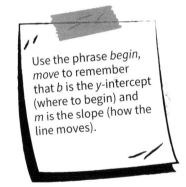

Use the phrase *begin, move* to remember that b is the y-intercept (where to begin) and m is the slope (how the line moves).

EXAMPLES

1. What is the slope of the line whose equation is
    $6x - 2y - 8 = 0$?

    Rearrange the equation into slope-intercept form by solving the equation for x:

    $6x - 2y - 8 = 0$

    Isolate $2y$ by subtracting $6x$ and adding 8 to both sides of the equation:

    $-2y = -6x + 8$

    "Undo" multiplication of -2 by y: divide both sides by -2:

    $y = \dfrac{-6x + 8}{-2}$

Simplify the fraction.

$y = 3x - 4$

The slope is 3, since it is the value attached to the x.

2. What is the equation of the following line?

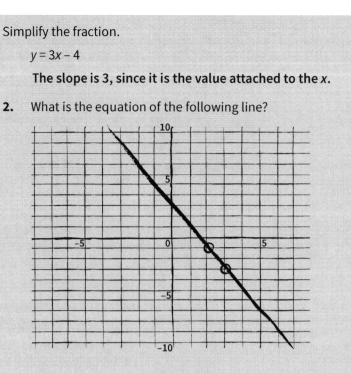

The y-intercept can be identified on the graph as $(0, 3)$. Thus, $b = 3$.

To find the slope, choose any two points and plug the values into the slope equation. The two points chosen here are $(2, -1)$ and $(3, -3)$.

$$m = \frac{(-3) - (-1)}{3 - 2} = \frac{-2}{1} = -2$$

Counting squares and verifying the line goes down 2 and over 1 to get from one point on the line to another point on the line gives the same result. Replace m with -2 and b with 3 in $y = mx + b$.

The equation is $y = -2x + 3$.

Building Equations

In word problems, it is often necessary to translate a verbal description of a relationship into a mathematical equation. No matter the problem, this process can be done using the same steps:

1. Read the problem carefully and identify what value needs to be solved for.

2. Identify the known and unknown quantities in the problem, and assign the unknown quantities a variable.

3. Create equations using the variables and known quantities.

4. Solve the equations.

5. Check the solution: does it answer the question asked in the problem? Does it make sense?

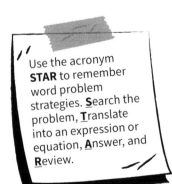

Use the acronym **STAR** to remember word problem strategies. **S**earch the problem, **T**ranslate into an expression or equation, **A**nswer, and **R**eview.

EXAMPLES

1. A school is holding a raffle to raise money. There is a $3.00 entry fee, and each ticket costs $5.00. If a student paid $28.00, how many tickets did he or she buy?

   The problem is asking for the number of tickets. First, identify the quantities:

   number of tickets = x

   cost per ticket = 5

   cost for x tickets = $5x$

   total cost = 28

   entry fee = 3

   Now, set up equations. The total cost for x tickets will be equal to the cost for x tickets plus the $3 entry fee:

   $5x + 3 = 28$

   Now solve the equation:

   $5x + 3 = 28$

   $5x = 25$

   $x = 5$

   The student bought 5 tickets.

2. Kelly is selling shirts for her school swim team. There are 2 prices: a student price and a non-student price. During the first week of the sale, Kelly raised $84 by selling 10 shirts to students and 4 shirts to non-students. She earned $185 in the second week by selling 20 shirts to students and 10 shirts to non-students. What is the student price for a shirt?

   The problem asks for the student price for shirts. Start by assigning variables:

   student price = s

   non-student price = n

   The number of shirts Kelly sold and the money she earned can be used to create 2 equations:

   $10s + 4n = 84$ (if 1 shirt costs s dollars, then 10 shirts cost $10s$ dollars, etc.)

   $20s + 10n = 185$

   Now, solve the system of equations using substitution. Since the question asks for the student price, the goal is to solve for s. Therefore, solve one of the equations for n so that when the expression is substituted for n, n will be eliminated and s will remain.

   $10s + 4n = 84$

   $10n = -20s + 185$

   $n = -2s + 18.5$

   $10s + 4(-2s + 18.5) = 84$

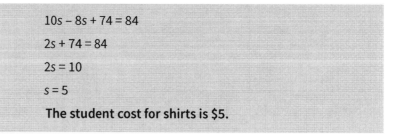

$10s - 8s + 74 = 84$

$2s + 74 = 84$

$2s = 10$

$s = 5$

The student cost for shirts is $5.

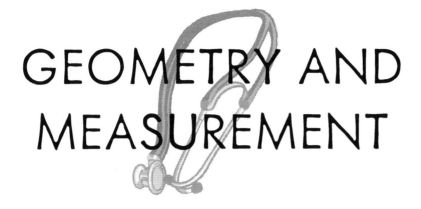

five

GEOMETRY AND MEASUREMENT

Units of Measurement

The standard units for the metric and American systems are shown below along with the prefixes used to express metric units.

Table 5.1. American and SI Units

DIMENSION	AMERICAN	SI
length	inch/foot/yard/mile	meter
mass	ounce/pound/ton	gram
volume	cup/pint/quart/gallon	liter
force	pound-force	newton
pressure	pound-force per square inch	pascal
work and energy	cal/British thermal unit	joule
temperature	Fahrenheit	kelvin
charge	faraday	coulomb

Table 5.2. Metric Prefixes

PREFIX	SYMBOL	MULTIPLICATION FACTOR
tera	T	1,000,000,000,000
giga	G	1,000,000,000
mega	M	1,000,000
kilo	k	1,000
hecto	h	100
deca	da	10
base unit	--	--
deci	d	0.1
centi	c	0.01
milli	m	0.001
micro	μ	0.0000001

Table 5.2. Metric Prefixes (continued)

Prefix	Symbol	Multiplication Factor
nano	n	0.0000000001
pico	p	0.0000000000001

Table 5.3. Conversion Factors

1 in. = 2.54 cm	1 lb. = 0.454 kg
1 yd. = 0.914 m	1 cal = 4.19 J
1 mi. = 1.61 km	$1°F = \frac{5}{9}(°F - 32°C)$
1 gal. = 3.785 L	$1 cm^3 = 1 mL$
1 oz. = 28.35 g	1 hr = 3600 s

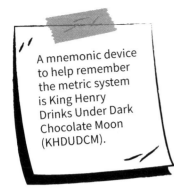

A mnemonic device to help remember the metric system is King Henry Drinks Under Dark Chocolate Moon (KHDUDCM).

Units can be converted within a single system or between systems. When converting from one unit to another unit, a CONVERSION FACTOR (a fraction used to convert a value with a unit into another unit) is used. For example, there are 2.54 centimeters in 1 inch, so the conversion factor from inches to centimeters is $\frac{2.54 \text{ centimeters}}{1 \text{ inch}}$.

To convert between units, multiply the original value by a conversion factor (or several if needed) so that the original units cancel, leaving the desired unit. Remember that the original value can be made into a fraction by placing it over 1.

$$\frac{3 \text{ inches}}{1} = \frac{2.54 \text{ centimeters}}{1 \text{ inch}} = 7.62 \text{ centimeters}$$

Units can be canceled (meaning they disappear from the expression) when they appear on the top and the bottom of a fraction. If the same unit appears in the top (or bottom) of both fractions, you probably need to flip the conversion factor.

EXAMPLES

1. Convert 4.25 kilometers to meters.

    $4.25 \text{ km} \left(\frac{1000 \text{ m}}{1 \text{ km}} \right) = 4250 \text{ m}$ (Because a meter is a smaller unit than a kilometer, multiply by 1000.)

2. Convert 12 feet to inches.

    $12 \text{ ft} \left(\frac{12 \text{ in}}{1 \text{ ft}} \right) = 144 \text{ in}$ (Since an inch is a smaller unit than a foot, multiply by 12 inches.)

Geometric Figures

Classifying Geometric Figures

GEOMETRIC FIGURES are shapes comprised of points, lines, or planes. A POINT is simply a location in space; it does not have any dimensional properties like length, area, or volume. A collection of points that extend infinitely in both directions is a LINE, and one that extends infinitely in only one direction is a RAY. A section of a line with a beginning and end point is a LINE SEGMENT. Lines, rays, and line segments are examples of ONE-DIMENSIONAL objects because they can only be measured in one dimension (length).

Figure 5.1. One-Dimensional Object

Lines, rays, and line segments can intersect to create ANGLES, which are measured in degrees or radians. Angles between zero and 90 degrees are ACUTE, and angles between 90 and 180 degrees are OBTUSE. An angle of exactly 90 degrees is a RIGHT ANGLE, and two lines that form right angles are PERPENDICULAR. Lines that do not intersect are described as PARALLEL.

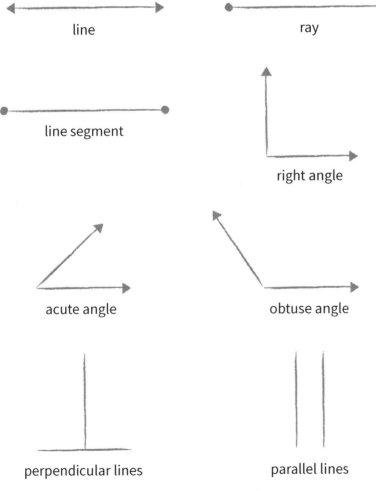

Figure 5.2. Lines and Angles

Two-dimensional objects can be measured in two dimensions—length and width. A PLANE is a two-dimensional object that extends infinitely in both directions. POLYGONS are two-dimensional shapes, such as triangles and squares, which have three or more straight sides. Regular polygons are polygons whose sides are all the same length.

Figure 5.3. Two-Dimensional Object

THREE-DIMENSIONAL objects, such as cubes, can be measured in three dimensions—length, width, and height.

Figure 5.4. Three-Dimensional Object

Calculating Geometric Quantities

The LENGTH, or distance from one point to another on an object, can be determined using a tape measure or a ruler. The size of the surface of a two-dimensional object is its AREA. Generally, the area of an object is its length times its width and is measured in square units. For example, if a window is 3 feet long and 2 feet wide, its area would be 6 ft^2.

The distance around a two dimensional figure is its PERIMETER, which can be found by adding the lengths of all the sides. The distance around a circle is referred to as its CIRCUMFERENCE.

Table 5.4. Area and Perimeter of Basic Shapes

SHAPE	EXAMPLE	AREA	PERIMETER
Triangle		$A = \frac{1}{2}bh$	$A = s_1 + s_2 + s_3$
Square		$A = s^2$	$A = 4s$
Rectangle		$A = l \times w$	$A = 2l + 2w$

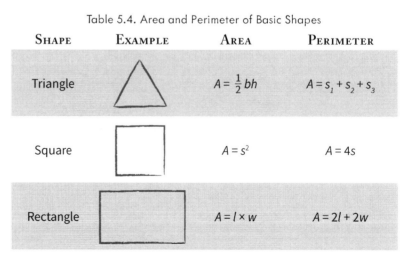

Shape	Example	Area	Perimeter
Parallelogram		$A = bh$	$A = s_1 + s_2 + s_3 + s_4$
Trapezoid		$A = \frac{1}{2}h(b_1 + b_2)$	$A = b_1 + b_2 + l_3 + l_4$
Rhombus		$A = \frac{1}{2}d_1 d_2$	$A = 4s$
Circle		$A = \pi r^2$	$A = 2\pi r$
Sector		$A = \frac{x°}{360°}(\pi r^2)$	$A = \frac{x°}{360°}(2\pi r)$

For the rectangle below, the area would be 8 m² because 2 m × 4 m = 8 m². The perimeter of the rectangle would be 12 meters because the sum of the length of all sides is 2 m + 4 m + 2 m + 4 m = 12 m.

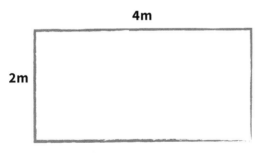

4m

2m

Figure 5.5. Perimeter

The SURFACE AREA of a three-dimensional object can be figured by adding the areas of all the sides. For example, the box below is 4 feet long, 3 feet wide, and 1 foot deep. The surface area is found by adding the areas of each face:

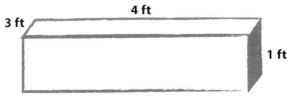

3 ft   **4 ft**   **1 ft**

Figure 5.6. Surface Area

- top: 4 ft × 3 ft = 12 ft²
- bottom: 4 ft × 3 ft = 12 ft²
- front: 4 ft × 1 ft = 4 ft²

- back: 4 ft × 1 ft = 4 ft^2
- right: 1 ft × 1 ft = 1 ft^2
- left: 1 ft × 1 ft = 1 ft^2

The TEAS will also ask test takers to find the perimeter and area of compound shapes, which will include parts of circles, squares, triangles, or other polygons joined together to create an irregular shape. For these types of problems, the first step is to divide the figure into shapes whose area (or perimeter) can easily be solved for. Then, solve each part separately and add (or subtract) the parts together for the final answer.

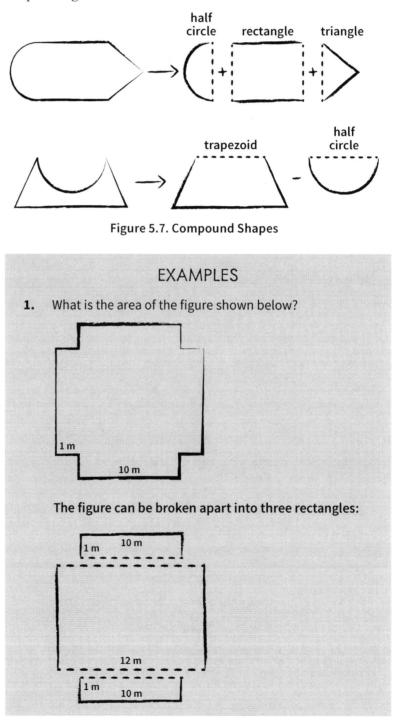

Figure 5.7. Compound Shapes

EXAMPLES

1. What is the area of the figure shown below?

The figure can be broken apart into three rectangles:

The area of each smaller rectangle is 1 m × 10 m = 10 m². The area of the larger rectangle is 10 m × 12 m = 120 m². Together, the area of the three shapes is 10 m² + 10 m² + 120 m² = 140 m²

2. What is the area of the shaded region in the figure below?

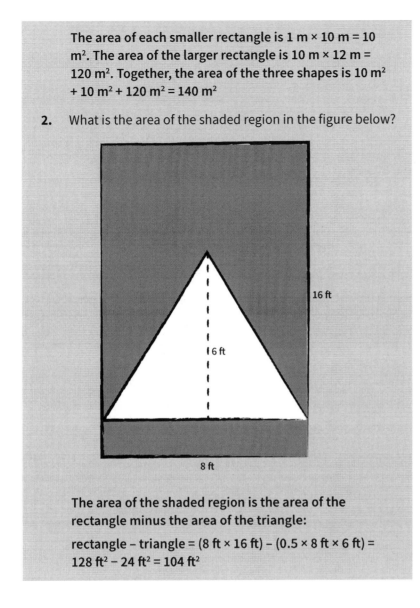

The area of the shaded region is the area of the rectangle minus the area of the triangle:

rectangle − triangle = (8 ft × 16 ft) − (0.5 × 8 ft × 6 ft) = 128 ft² − 24 ft² = 104 ft²

Data Presentation

Data can be presented in a variety of ways. In addition to a simple table, there are a number of different graphs and charts that can be used to visually represent data. The most appropriate depends on the data being displayed.

BOX PLOTS (also called box and whisker plots) show data using the median, range, and outliers of a data set. They provide a helpful visual guide, showing how data is distributed around the median. In the example below, 81 is the median and the range is 0 – 100, or 100.

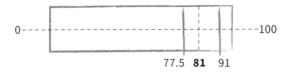

Figure 5.8. Box Plot

BAR GRAPHS use bars of different lengths to compare data. The independent variable on a bar graph is grouped into categories such as months, flavors, or locations, and the dependent variable will be a quantity. Thus, comparing the length of bars provides a visual guide to the relative amounts in each category. DOUBLE BAR GRAPHS show more than one data set on the same set of axes.

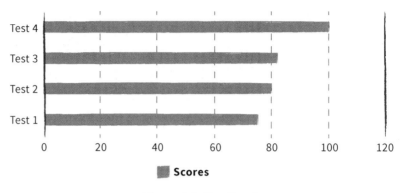

Figure 5.9. Bar Graph

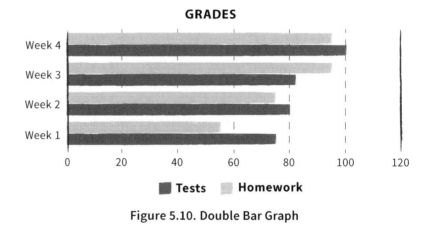

Figure 5.10. Double Bar Graph

HISTOGRAMS similarly use bars to compare data, but the independent variable is a continuous variable that has been "binned" or divided into categories. For example, the time of day can be broken down into 8:00 a.m. to 12:00 p.m., 12:00 p.m. to 4:00 p.m., and so on. Usually (but not always), a gap is included between the bars of a bar graph but not a histogram.

DOT PLOTS display the frequency of a value or event data graphically using dots, and thus can be used to observe the distribution of a data set. Typically, a value or category is listed on the x-axis, and the number of times that value appears in the data set is represented by a line of vertical dots. Dot plots make it easy to see which values occur most often.

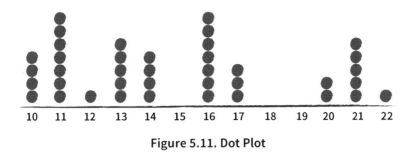

Figure 5.11. Dot Plot

SCATTER PLOTS use points to show relationships between two variables which can be plotted as coordinate points. One variable describes a position on the *x*-axis, and the other a point on the *y*-axis. Scatter plots can suggest relationships between variables. For example, both variables might increase, or one may increase when the other decreases.

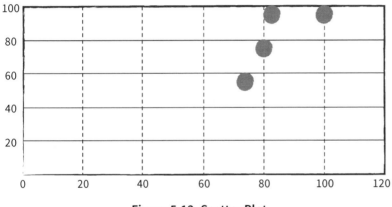

Figure 5.12. Scatter Plot

LINE GRAPHS show changes in data by connecting points on a scatter graph using a line. These graphs will often measure time on the *x*-axis and are used to show trends in the data, such as temperature changes over a day or school attendance throughout the year.

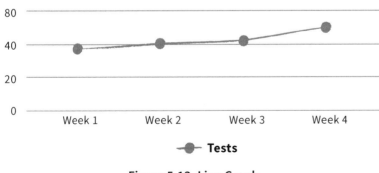

Figure 5.13. Line Graph

DOUBLE LINE GRAPHS present two sets of data on the same set of axes.

GO ON

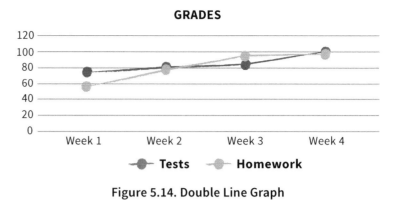

GRADES

Figure 5.14. Double Line Graph

Circle graphs (also called pie charts) are used to show parts of a whole: the "pie" is the whole, and each "slice" represents a percentage or part of the whole.

TESTS

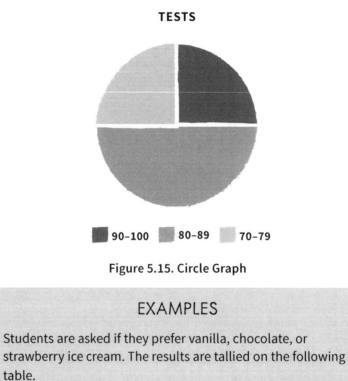

■ 90–100   ■ 80–89   ▨ 70–79

Figure 5.15. Circle Graph

EXAMPLES

Students are asked if they prefer vanilla, chocolate, or strawberry ice cream. The results are tallied on the following table.

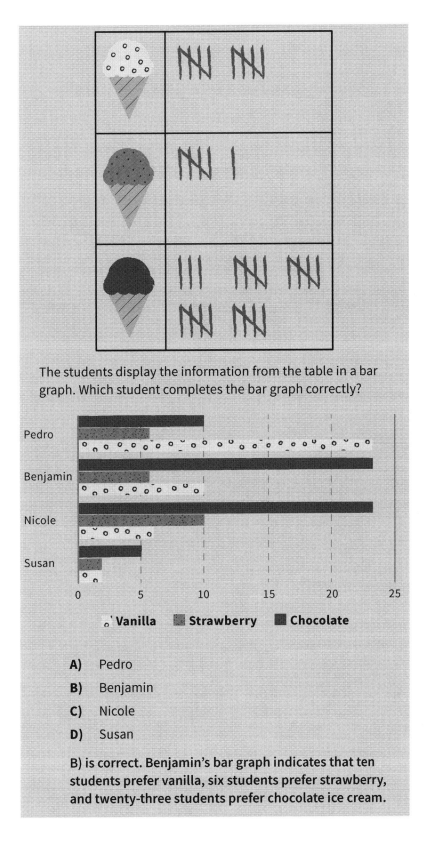

The students display the information from the table in a bar graph. Which student completes the bar graph correctly?

A) Pedro

B) Benjamin

C) Nicole

D) Susan

B) is correct. Benjamin's bar graph indicates that ten students prefer vanilla, six students prefer strawberry, and twenty-three students prefer chocolate ice cream.

Statistics

STATISTICS is the study of data. Analyzing data requires using **MEASURES OF CENTER** (mean, median, and mode) to identify trends or patterns.

The MEAN is the average; it is determined by adding all outcomes and then dividing by the total number of outcomes. For example, the average of the data set {16, 19, 19, 25, 27, 29, 75} is equal to $\frac{16 + 19 + 19 + 25 + 27 + 29 + 75}{7} = \frac{210}{7} = 30$.

The MEDIAN is the number in the middle when the data set is arranged in order from least to greatest. For example, in the data set {16, 19, 19, **25**, 27, 29, 75}, the median is 25. When a data set contains an even number of values, finding the median requires averaging the two middle values. In the data set {75, 80, 82, 100}, the two numbers in the middle are 80 and 82. Consequently, the median will be the average of these two values: $\frac{80 + 82}{2} = 81$.

Finally, the MODE is the most frequent outcome in a data set. In the set {16, 19, 19, 25, 27, 29, 75}, the mode is 19 because it occurs twice, which is more than any of the other numbers. If several values appear an equal, and most frequent, number of times, both values are considered the mode.

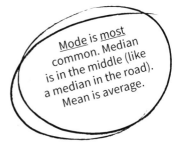

Mode is most common. Median is in the middle (like a median in the road). Mean is average.

Other useful indicators include range and outliers. The RANGE is the difference between the highest and the lowest number in a data set. For example, the range of the set {16, 19, 19, 25, 27, 29, 75} is 75 − 16 = 59.

OUTLIERS, or data points that are much different from other data points, should be noted as they can skew the central tendency. In the data set {16, 19, 19, 25, 27, 29, 75}, the value 75 is far outside the other values and raises the value of the mean. Without the outlier, the mean is much closer to the other data points.

- $\frac{16 + 19 + 19 + 25 + 27 + 29 + 75}{7} = \frac{210}{7} = 30$
- $\frac{16 + 19 + 19 + 25 + 27 + 29}{6} = \frac{135}{6} = 22.5$

Generally, the median is a better indicator of a central tendency if outliers are present to skew the mean.

Trends in a data set can also be seen by graphing the data as a dot plot. The distribution of the data can then be described based on the shape of the graph. A SYMMETRIC distribution looks like two mirrored halves, while a SKEWED distribution is weighted more heavily toward the right or the left. Note the direction of the skew describes the side of the graph with fewer data points. In a UNIFORM data set, the points are distributed evenly along the graph.

A symmetric or skewed distribution may have peaks, or sets of data points that appear more frequently. A UNIMODAL distribution has one peak while a BIMODAL distribution has two peaks. A normal (or bell-shaped) distribution is a special symmetric, unimodal graph with a specific distribution of data points.

EXAMPLES

1. Which of the following is the mean of the data set?

   14, 18, 11, 28, 23, 14

   A) 11

   B) 14

   C) 18

   D) 28

   C) is correct. The mean is the average:

   $$\frac{14 + 18 + 11 + 28 + 23 + 14}{6} = \frac{108}{6} = 18$$

2. Which of the following best describes the distribution of the graph?

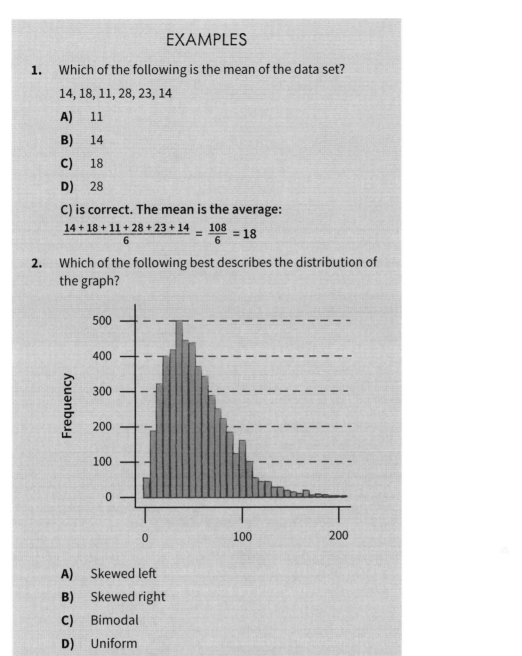

   A) Skewed left

   B) Skewed right

   C) Bimodal

   D) Uniform

   B) is correct. The graph is skewed right because there are fewer data points on the right half.

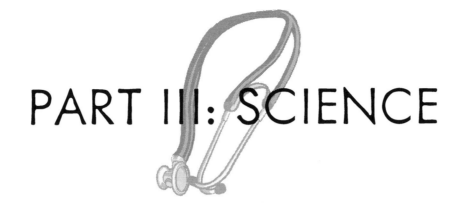

PART III: SCIENCE

six

ANATOMY AND PHYSIOLOGY

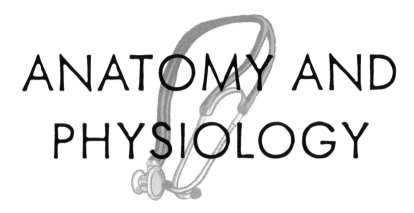

General Anatomy and Physiology

The Biological Hierarchy

Organisms are living things consisting of at least one cell, which is the smallest unit of life that can reproduce on its own. Unicellular organisms, such as the amoeba, are made up of only one cell, while multicellular organisms are comprised of many cells. In a multicellular organism, the cells are grouped together into TISSUES, and these tissues are grouped into ORGANS, which perform a specific function. The heart, for example, is the organ that pumps blood throughout the body. Organs are further grouped into ORGAN SYSTEMS, such as the digestive or respiratory systems.

Anatomical Terminology

Learning anatomy requires an understanding of the terminology used to describe the location and morphology of a particular structure. Anatomical science uses common terms to describe spatial relationships, often in pairs of opposites. These terms often refer to the position of a structure in an organism that is upright with respect to its environment (e.g. in its typical orientation while moving forward).

The terms SUPERIOR, meaning *above* in this context, and INFERIOR, meaning *below*, are probably the simplest to grasp due to their colloquial usage. For example, the anatomical description of a human face to an individual that had never seen one might describe the eyes as being superior to the nose in anatomical positioning.

A system is a collection of interconnected parts that make up a complex whole with defined boundaries. Systems may be closed, meaning nothing passes in or out of them, or open, meaning they have inputs and outputs. Organ systems are open and will have a number of inputs and outputs.

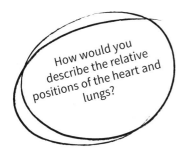
ANTERIOR usually refers to a structure that is in front of another reference point, with **POSTERIOR** meaning the opposite. In humans, the eyes are anterior with respect to the ears; conversely, the ears are posterior with respect to the eyes.

DORSAL refers to a structure closer to the back of an object, with **VENTRAL** being its opposite. A useful mnemonic for this may be the dorsal and ventral fins commonly described on fish, or the fact the spine is found dorsally in humans whereas the stomach is more ventral.

Features nearer to the middle of a structure are referred to as being **MEDIAL**, whereas those further from the center or closer to the outer boundaries are referred to as being **LATERAL**.

Finally, **PROXIMAL** describes a structure that is closer, and **DISTAL** further away. The index finger is more proximal to the hand than is the elbow, which is more distal to the hand in comparison to the location of the index finger.

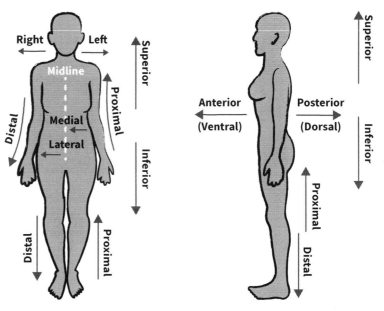

Figure 6.1. Anatomy Terminology

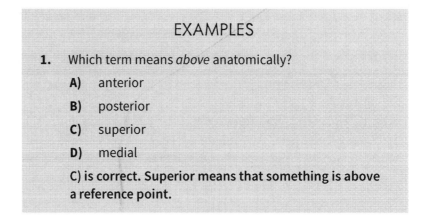

EXAMPLES

1. Which term means *above* anatomically?

    A) anterior

    B) posterior

    C) superior

    D) medial

    C) is correct. Superior means that something is above a reference point.

The Respiratory System

Mammalian cells require oxygen for glucose metabolism and release carbon dioxide as a byproduct. This process requires constant gas exchange between the human body and the environment to replenish the oxygen supply and remove carbon dioxide. This exchange is accomplished through the efforts of the **RESPIRATORY SYSTEM**, in which powerful muscles force oxygen-rich air into the lungs and carbon dioxide-rich air out of the body.

Gas exchange takes place in the **LUNGS**. Humans have two lungs, a right and a left, with the right being slightly larger than the left due to the heart's placement in the left side of the chest cavity. The right lung has three **LOBES**, and the left has two. The lungs are surrounded by a thick membrane called the **PLEURA**.

Air enters the body through the mouth or nasal cavity and passes through the **TRACHEA** (sometimes called the windpipe) and into the two bronchi, each of which leads to one lung. Within the lung, the bronchi branch into smaller passageways called **BRON-CHIOLES** and then terminate in sac-like structures called **ALVEOLI**,

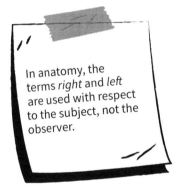

In anatomy, the terms *right* and *left* are used with respect to the subject, not the observer.

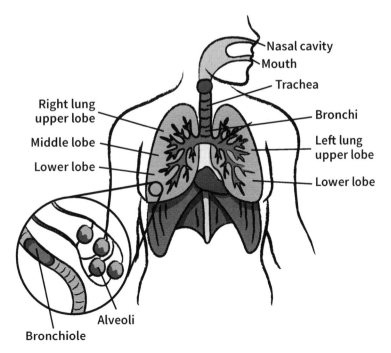

Figure 6.2. The Respiratory System

which is where gas exchange between the air and the capillaries occurs. The large surface area of the alveoli allows for efficient exchange of gases through diffusion (movement of particles from areas of high to low concentration). Alveoli are covered in a layer of SURFACTANT, which lubricates the sacs and prevents the lungs from collapsing.

The heart pumps deoxygenated blood into the lungs via the PULMONARY ARTERY. This blood is oxygenated in the alveoli and then delivered back into the heart by the PULMONARY VEINS for distribution to the body.

The DIAPHRAGM contributes to the activity of ventilation—the process of inhalation and exhalation. The contraction of the diaphragm creates a vacuum, forcing air into the lungs. Relaxation of the diaphragm compresses the lungs, forcing carbon dioxide-enriched gas out in exhalation. The amount of air breathed in and out is the TIDAL VOLUME, and the RESIDUAL CAPACITY is the small volume of air left in the lungs after exhalation.

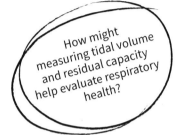
How might measuring tidal volume and residual capacity help evaluate respiratory health?

Pathologies of the Respiratory System

The body's critical and constant need for the exchange of carbon dioxide for oxygen makes the pulmonary system a locus of many serious diseases. Broadly, lung disease resulting in the continual restriction of airflow is known as CHRONIC OBSTRUCTIVE PULMONARY DISEASE (COPD), with the destruction of alveoli in particular resulting in EMPHYSEMA. ASTHMA is a common condition restricting airflow, in which the airways are compromised due to a dysfunctional immune response. Asthma can be caused by a range of environmental factors, including pollution and smoking, while COPD is mostly a result of chronic smoking.

The system is also prone to RESPIRATORY TRACT INFECTIONS, with upper respiratory tract infections affecting air inputs in the nose and throat and lower respiratory tract infections affecting the lungs and their immediate pulmonary inputs. Viral infections of the respiratory system include influenza and the common cold; bacterial infections include tuberculosis and pertussis (whooping cough). PNEUMONIA, which affects alveoli, is a bacterial or viral infection that is often seen in people whose respiratory system has been weakened by other conditions.

EXAMPLES

1. Which of the following contains deoxygenated blood?
   A) alveoli
   B) pulmonary artery
   C) pulmonary vein
   D) diaphragm

The Cardiovascular System

The cardiovascular system circulates blood throughout the body. Blood carries a wide range of molecules necessary for the body to function, including nutrients, wastes, hormones, and gases. Blood is broken into a number of different parts. Red blood cells called HEMOGLOBIN transport oxygen, and white blood cells circulate as part of the immune system. Both red and white blood cells are suspended in a fluid called PLASMA, in which are dissolved the other molecules transported by the blood.

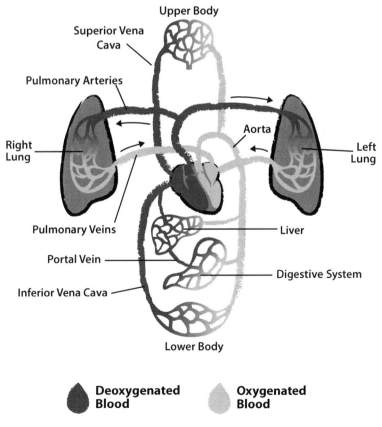

Figure 6.3 Circulatory System

Blood is circulated by a muscular organ called the HEART. The circulatory system includes two closed loops. In the pulmonary loop, deoxygenated blood leaves the heart and travels to the lungs, where it loses carbon dioxide and becomes rich in oxygen. The oxygenated blood then returns to the heart, which pumps it through the systemic loop. The systemic loop delivers oxygen to the rest of the body and returns deoxygenated blood to the heart. The pumping action of the heart is regulated primarily by two neurological nodes, the SINOATRIAL and ATRIOVENTRICULAR NODES, whose electrical activity sets the rhythm of the heart.

Deoxygenated blood from the body enters the heart via the RIGHT ATRIUM. It then passes through the TRICUSPID valve into the RIGHT VENTRICLE and is pumped out to the lungs. Oxygenated blood returns from the blood into the LEFT ATRIUM. It then passes through the MITRAL VALVE into the LEFT VENTRICLE and is pumped out to the body through the AORTA. The contraction of the heart during this process is called SYSTOLE, and the relaxation of the heart is DIASTOLE.

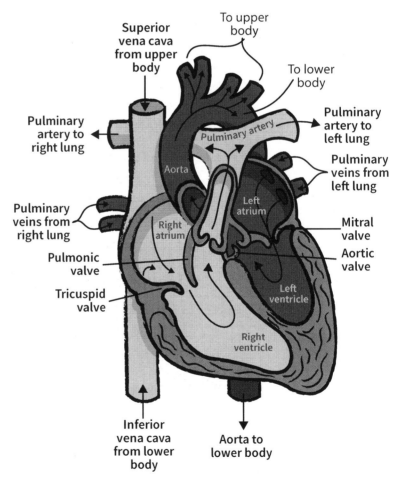

Figure 6.4. The Heart

Blood is carried through the body in a system of blood vessels. Oxygenated blood leaves the heart in large vessels called ARTERIES, which branch into smaller and smaller vessels. The smallest vessels, CAPILLARIES, are where the exchange of molecules between blood and cells takes place. Deoxygenated blood returns to the heart in VEINS.

The Lymphatic System

The LYMPHATIC SYSTEM is an open circulatory system that functions alongside the cardiovascular system. It facilitates the movement of substances between cells and the blood by removing interstitial fluid (the fluid between cells). It also plays an important role in the immune system by circulating white blood cells. The system is composed of LYMPHATIC VESSELS that carry LYMPH, a clear fluid containing lymphocytes and waste products. Lymph passes through LYMPH NODES, which are collections of tissue rich in white blood cells. It is then returned to the circulatory system through the veins near the heart.

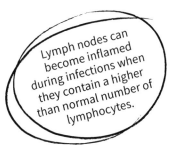

Lymph nodes can become inflamed during infections when they contain a higher than normal number of lymphocytes.

Pathologies of the Cardiovascular System

The cardiovascular system is subject to a number of pathologies. In a HEART ATTACK, blood flow to part of the heart is stopped, causing damage to the heart muscle. An irregular heartbeat, called an ARRHYTHMIA, is caused by disruptions with the electrical signals in the heart. Many arrhythmias can be treated—with a pacemaker, for example—or do not cause any symptoms.

Problems with blood vessels include ATHEROSCLEROSIS, in which white blood cells and plaque build up in arteries, and HYPERTENSION, or high blood pressure. In a stroke, blood flow is blocked in the brain, resulting in damage to brain cells.

EXAMPLES

1. The mitral valve transports blood between which of the following two regions of the heart?

    A) aorta and left atrium

    B) aorta and right atrium

    C) right atrium and right ventricle

    D) left atrium and left ventricle

    D) is correct. These two structures form a junction at the mitral valve.

2. Which of the following supplies blood to the lower body?

    A) superior vena cava

    B) inferior vena cava

    C) iliac artery

    D) aortic arch

3. Which of the following electrically signals the heart to pump?

    A) sinoatrial node

    B) aorta

    C) mitral valve

    D) left ventricle

    A) is correct. The sinoatrial and atrioventricular nodes electrically stimulate the heart to pump.

The Nervous System

The nervous system is made up of two distinct parts: the central nervous system (brain and spinal cord) and the peripheral nervous system. However, the fundamental physiological principles underlying both systems are similar. In both systems, NEURONS communicate electrically and chemically with one another along pathways. These pathways allow the nervous system as a whole to conduct its incredibly broad array of functions, from motor control and sensory perception to complex thinking and emotions.

Nerve Cells

Neurons, a.k.a. nerve cells, have several key anatomical features that contribute to their specialized functions. These cells typically contain an AXON, a long projection from the cell that sends information over a distance. These cells also have DENDRITES, which are long, branching extensions of the cell that receive information from neighboring cells. The number of dendrites and the extent of their branching varies widely, distinguishing the various types of these cells.

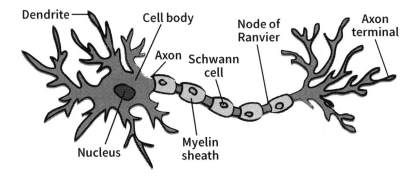

Figure 6.5. Nerve Cell

Neurons and nerve cells do not touch; instead, communication occurs across a specialized gap called a SYNAPSE. The chemicals that facilitate communication across synapses are known as NEUROTRANSMITTERS, and include serotonin and dopamine. Communication occurs when electrical signals cause the AXON TERMINAL to release neurotransmitters.

Nerve cells are accompanied by glia, or supporting cells, that surround the cell and provide support, protection, and nutrients. In the peripheral nervous system, the primary glial cell is a SCHWANN CELL. Schwann cells secrete a fatty substance called MYELIN that wraps around the neuron and allows much faster transmission of the electrical signal the neuron is sending. Gaps in the myelin sheath are called nodes of Ranvier.

Nerve cell signaling is controlled by moving ions across the cell membrane to maintain an electric potential. Depolarizing the cell, or lowering the electric potential, triggers the release of neurotransmitters.

The Central Nervous System

The central nervous system, which includes the brain and spinal cord, is responsible for arguably the body's most complex and abstract functions, including cognition, emotion, and behavioral regulation.

In general, the brain is organized into lobes that each carry out a broad, common function. For example, the processing of visual information occurs in the OCCIPITAL LOBE, and the TEMPORAL LOBE is involved in language comprehension and emotional associations. In addition to its organization by lobes and structures, regions of the brain are also designated by myelination status: WHITE MATTER regions are myelinated and GRAY MATTER regions are unmyelinated. Brain structures in the cerebral cortex (the outermost brain layer) form a convoluted pattern of GYRI (ridges) and SULCI (valleys) that maximize the ratio of surface area to volume.

Alzheimer's disease, which causes dementia, is the result of damaged neurons in the cerebral cortex, the area of the brain responsible for higher order functions like information processing and language.

The Peripheral Nervous System

The peripheral nervous system, which includes all the nerve cells outside the brain and spinal cord, has one main function and that is to communicate between the CNS and the rest of the body.

The peripheral nervous system is further divided into two systems. The AUTOMATIC NERVOUS SYSTEM (ANS) is the part of the peripheral nervous system that controls involuntary bodily functions such as digestion, respiration, and heart rate. These aspects of the automatic nervous system are controlled by the hypothalamus. The adrenal glands control the "fight or flight" bodily response that is also part of the automatic nervous system.

The second part of the peripheral nervous system, called the somatic nervous system, controls sensory information and motor control. Generally, nerve cells can be divided into two types. AFFERENT (sensory) cells relay messages to the central nervous system, and EFFERENT (motor) cells carry messages to the muscles. In the motor nervous system, signals from the brain travel down the spinal cord before exiting and communicating with motor nerve cells, which synapse on muscle fibers at NEUROMUSCULAR JUNCTIONS. Because individuals can control the movement of skeletal muscle, this part of the nervous system is considered voluntary.

Some REFLEXES, or automatic response to stimuli, are able to occur rapidly by bypassing the brain altogether. In a REFLEX ARC, a signal is sent from the peripheral nervous system to the spinal cord, which then sends a signal directly to a motor cells, causing movement.

The "fight or flight" reaction includes accelerated breathing and heart rate, dilation of blood vessels in muscles, release of energy molecules for use by muscles, relaxation of the bladder, and slowing or stopping movement in the upper digestive tract.

EXAMPLES

1. Which of the following is not controlled by the automatic nervous system?

   A) walking

   B) blinking

   C) breathing

   D) sexual arousal

   A) is correct. Walking is a voluntary action not controlled by the automatic nervous system.

2. Which of the following is the part of a nerve cell that receives information?

   A) axon

   B) dendrite

   C) Schwann cell

   D) myelin

   B) is correct. Dendrites receive information in nerve cells.

The Gastrointestinal System

Fueling the biological systems mentioned previously is the digestive system. The digestive system is essentially a continuous tube in which food is processed. During digestion, the body extracts necessary nutrients and biological fuels and isolates waste to be discarded.

The breakdown of food into its constituent parts begins as soon as it is put into the mouth. Enzymes in SALIVA such as salivary amylase begin breaking down food, particularly starch, as mastication helps prepare food for swallowing and subsequent digestion. Food from this point is formed into a BOLUS that travels down the esophagus, aided by a process called PERISTALSIS, rhythmic contractions that move the partially-digested food towards the stomach. Upon reaching the STOMACH, food encounters a powerful acid (hydrochloric acid, produced by the stomach itself), which aids the breakdown of food into its absorbable components.

The burning sensation called heartburn occurs when gastric acid from the stomach travels up the esophagus, often as a result of relaxation of the lower esophageal sphincter. This acid can damage the lining of the esophagus.

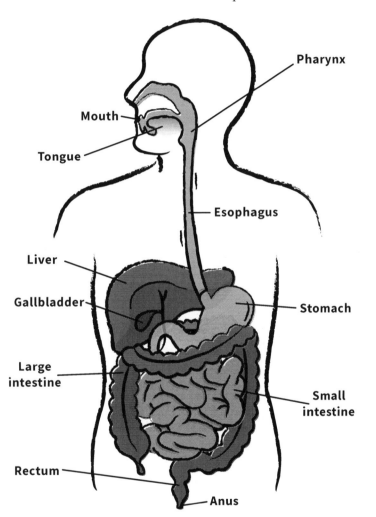

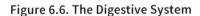

Figure 6.6. The Digestive System

The human body derives fuel primarily from three sources: proteins, sugars, and fats (lipids). Enzymes break proteins down into their constituent amino acids to produce new proteins for the body. Carbohydrates are broken down enzymatically if necessary and used for metabolism. Fats are broken down into constituent fatty acids and glycerol for a number of uses, including dense nutritional energy storage. Digestion of fat requires BILE acids produced by the LIVER; bile is stored in the GALL BLADDER.

The stomach produces a semifluid mass of partially digested food called CHYME that then passes into the SMALL INTESTINE, where nutrients are absorbed into the bloodstream. This occurs through MUCOSAL CELLS in the lining of the intestine. The small intestine itself has three major segments. Proximal to the stomach is the DUODENUM, which combines digestive substances from the liver and pancreas; next is the JEJUNUM, the primary site of nutrient absorption; finally, the ILEUM absorbs remaining nutrients and moves the remaining matter into the large intestine. The LARGE INTESTINE (also called the colon) absorbs water from the waste, which then passes into the RECTUM and out of the body through the ANUS.

Pathologies of the Digestive System

The digestive system is prone to several illnesses of varying severity. Commonly, gastrointestinal distress is caused by an acute infection (bacterial or viral) affecting the lining of the digestive system. A resulting immune response triggers the body, as an adaptive measure, to void the contents of the digestive system in order to purge the infection. Chronic gastrointestinal disorders include IRRITABLE BOWEL SYNDROME (the causes of which are largely unknown) and CROHN'S DISEASE, an inflammatory bowel disorder with an immune-related etiology.

EXAMPLES

1. Which absorbs nutrients into the bloodstream?
   A) colon
   B) duodenum
   C) mucosal cells
   D) enzymes

   C) is correct. Mucosal cells in the small intestine absorb nutrients into the bloodstream.

2. Which initiates the breakdown of carbohydrates?
   A) salivary amylase
   B) stomach acid
   C) bile salts
   D) peristalsis

   A) is correct. Salivary amylase in the mouth begins the breakdown of carbohydrates.

The Skeletal System

The skeletal system is composed of tissue called BONE that helps with movement, provides support for organs, and synthesizes blood cells. The outer layer of bone is composed of a matrix made of collagen and minerals that gives bones their strength and rigidity. The matrix is formed from functional units called OSTEONS that include layers of compact bone called LAMELLAE. The lamellae surround a cavity called the HAVERSIAN CANAL, which houses the bone's blood supply. These canals are in turn connected to the PERIOSTEUM, the bone's outermost membrane, by another series of channels called VOLKMANN'S CANALS.

Within osteons are blood cells called OSTEOBLASTS, mononucleate cells that produce bone tissue. When the bone tissue hardens around these cells, the cells are known as OSTEOCYTES, and the space they occupy within the bone tissue is known as LACUNAE. The lacunae are connected by a series of channels called CANALICULI. OSTEOCLASTS, a third type of bone cell, are responsible for breaking down bone tissue. They are located on the surface of bones and help balance the body's calcium levels by degrading bone to release stored calcium. The fourth type of bone cell, LINING CELLS are flatted osteoblasts that protect the bone and also help balance calcium levels.

Within the hard outer layer of bone is the spongy layer called TRABECULAE. Within this layer is the bone marrow, which houses cells that produce red blood cells in a process called HEMATOPOIESIS. Bone marrow also produces many of the lymphocytes that play an important role in the immune system.

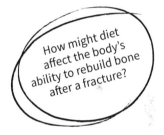

How might diet affect the body's ability to rebuild bone after a fracture?

Bones are divided into four main categories. LONG BONES, such as the femur and humerus, are longer than they are wide. SHORT BONES, in contrast, are wider than they are long. These include the clavicle and carpals. FLAT BONES are wide and flat, and usually provide protection. Examples of flat bones include the bones of the skull, pelvis, and rib cage. IRREGULAR BONES, as the name suggests, have an irregular shape that doesn't fit into the other categories. These bones include the vertebrae and bones of the jaw.

GO ON

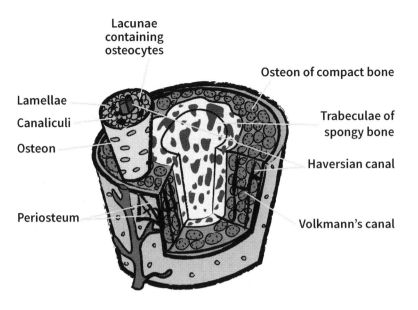

Figure 6.7. Bone Structure

Bones are held together (articulated) at JOINTS by connective tissue called LIGAMENTS. Joints can be classified based on the tissue that connects the bone. FIBROUS JOINTS are connected by dense, collagen-rich fibers, while CARTILAGINOUS JOINTS are joined by special tissue called HYALINE CARTILAGE. Cartilage is more flexible than bone but denser than muscles. In addition to joining together bone, it also helps hold open passage ways and provides support in structures like the nose and ears. The third type of joint, SYNOVIAL

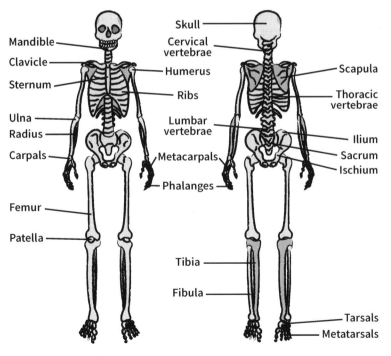

Figure 6.8. The Skeletal System

JOINTS, are joined by synovial fluid, which lubricates the joint and allows for movement. Bones are also joined to muscles by connective tissue called TENDONS.

Pathologies of the Skeletal System

Important pathologies of the skeletal system include OSTEOPOROSIS, which occurs when minerals are leached from the bone, making bones more likely to break. Broken bones can also be caused by BRITTLE BONE DISEASE, which results from a genetic defect that affects collagen production. Joint pain can be caused by OSTEOARTHRITIS, which is the breakdown of cartilage in joints, and RHEUMATOID ARTHRITIS, which is an autoimmune disease that affects synovial membranes.

EXAMPLES

1. Which type of cell is responsible for the degradation of bone tissue?

    A) osteoclasts

    B) osteoblasts

    C) osteocytes

    D) lining cells

    A) is correct. Osteoclasts break down and absorb bone tissue.

2. Which of the following is a flat bone?

    A) tarsals

    B) radius

    C) sternum

    D) mandible

    C) is correct. The sternum is a flat bone.

The Muscular System

The muscular system is composed of MUSCLES that move the body, support bodily functions, and circulate blood. The human body contains three types of muscles. SKELETAL MUSCLES are voluntarily controlled and attach to the skeleton to allow movement in the body. SMOOTH MUSCLES are involuntary, meaning they cannot be consciously controlled. Smooth muscles are found in many organs and structures, including the esophagus, stomach, intestines, blood vessels, bladder, and bronchi. Finally, CARDIAC MUSCLES, found only in the heart, are the involuntary muscles that contract the heart in order to pump blood through the body.

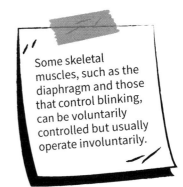

Some skeletal muscles, such as the diaphragm and those that control blinking, can be voluntarily controlled but usually operate involuntarily.

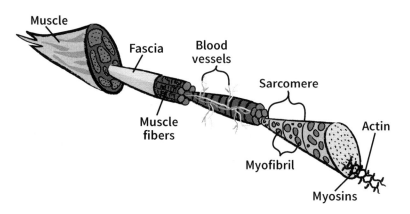

Figure 6.9. Structure of Skeletal Muscle

Muscle is composed of two proteins: ACTIN (thin filaments) and MYOSIN (thick filaments). These proteins are arranged in a lattice structure. When the muscle receives a signal from a motor neuron, the actin and myosin slide past each other to CONTRACT, or shorten, the muscle. When they return to their resting position, the muscle is RELAXED. The process of contraction requires the energy molecule ATP.

In skeletal and cardiac muscle, actin and myosin are bundled into SARCOMERES, which are the building blocks of the tubular muscle fibers called MYOFIBRILS. The sarcomeres appear as alternating dark and light bands under a light microscope.

Pathologies of the Muscular System

Injuries to muscle can impede movement and cause pain. When muscle fibers are overstretched, the resulting MUSCLE STRAIN can cause pain, stiffness, and bruising. Muscle fibers can also be weakened by diseases, as with MUSCULAR DYSTROPHY (MD). MD is a genetically inherited condition that results in progressive muscle wasting, which limits movement and can cause respiratory and cardiovascular difficulties.

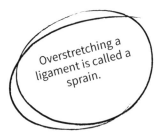

Overstretching a ligament is called a sprain.

EXAMPLES

1. Which of the following is controlled by skeletal muscle?

    A) digestion

    B) walking

    C) blood flow

    D) uterine contractions

    B) is correct. Walking is a voluntary action controlled by skeletal muscles.

The Immune System

The human immune system protects the body against bacteria and viruses that cause disease. The system is composed of two parts. The INNATE system includes nonspecific defenses that work against a wide range of infectious agents. This system includes both physical barriers that keep out foreign particles and organisms along with specific cells that attack invaders that move past barriers. The second part of the immune system is the ADAPTIVE immune system, which "learns" to respond only to specific invaders.

Table 6.1. Lines of Defense in the Immune System

1. EXTERNAL BARRIERS	skin, enzymes, mucus, earwax, native bacteria
2. THE INNATE RESPONSE	inflammation, eukocytes (white blood cells), antimicrobial peptides, natural killer lymphocytes, interferon
3. THE ADAPTIVE RESPONSE	helper T-cells, cytotoxic T-cells, B-cells, memory B-cells

The Innate Immune System

The first line of defense in the immune system are barriers to entry. The most prominent is the SKIN, which leaves few openings for an infection-causing agent to enter. Bodily orifices exhibit other methods for preventing infection. The mouth is saturated with native bacteria that dominate the resources in the microenvironment, making it inhospitable to invading bacteria. In addition, enzymes in the mouth create a hostile environment for foreign organisms. The urethra flushes away potentially invasive microorganisms mechanically through the outflow of urine, while the vagina maintains a consistently low pH, deterring potential infections. The eyes and nose constantly produce and flush away tears and MUCUS, which trap pathogens before they can replicate and infect. Similarly, EARWAX serves as an additional barrier to entry.

Pathogens do occasionally breach these barriers and arrive within the body, where they attempt to replicate and cause an infection. When this occurs, the body mounts a number of nonspecific responses. The body's initial response is INFLAMMATION: infected cells release signaling molecules indicating that an infection has occurred, which causes increased blood flow to the area. This increase in blood flow includes the increased presence of WHITE BLOOD CELLS, also called LEUKOCYTES. The most common type of leukocyte found at sites of inflammation are NEUTROPHILS, which engulf and destroy invaders.

Other innate responses include ANTIMICROBIAL PEPTIDES, which destroy bacteria by interfering with the functions of their membranes or DNA, and NATURAL KILLER LYMPHOCYTES, which respond to virus-infected cells. Because they can recognize damaged cells with the presence of antibodies, they are important in early defense against bacterial infection. In addition, infected cells may release INTERFERON, which causes nearby cells to increase their defenses.

The Adaptive Immune System

The adaptive immune system is able to recognize molecules called ANTIGENS on the surface of pathogens to which the system has previously been exposed. Antigens are displayed on the surface of cells by the MAJOR HISTOCOMPATIBILITY COMPLEX (MHC), which can display either "self" proteins from their own cells or proteins from pathogens. In an ANTIGEN-PRESENTING CELL, the MHC on the cell's surface displays a particular antigen, which is recognized by HELPER T-CELLS. These cells produce a signal (cytokines) that activates CYTOTOXIC T-CELLS, which then destroy any cell that displays the antigen.

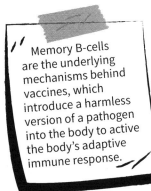

Memory B-cells are the underlying mechanisms behind vaccines, which introduce a harmless version of a pathogen into the body to active the body's adaptive immune response.

The presence of antigens also activates B-CELLS, which rapidly multiply to create PLASMA CELLS, which in turn release ANTIBODIES. Antibodies will bind only to specific antigens, and in turn result in the destruction of the infected cell. Some interfere directly with the function of the cell, while others draw the attention of macrophages. MEMORY B-CELLS are created during infection. These cells "remember" the antigen that their parent cells responded to, allowing them to respond more quickly if the infection appears again.

Together, T- and B-cells are known as LYMPHOCYTES. T-cells are produced in the thymus, while B-cells mature in bone marrow. These cells circulate through the lymphatic system.

Pathologies of the Immune System

The immune system itself can be pathological. The immune system of individuals with an AUTOIMMUNE DISEASE will attack healthy tissues, as is the case in lupus, psoriasis, and multiple sclerosis. The immune system may also overreact to harmless particles, a condition known as an ALLERGY. Some infections will attack the immune system itself. HUMAN IMMUNODEFICIENCY VIRUS (HIV) attacks helper T-cells, eventually causing ACQUIRED IMMUNODEFICIENCY SYNDROME (AIDS), which allows opportunistic infections to overrun the body.

EXAMPLES

1. Which of the following is NOT part of the innate immune system?

   A) interferon

   B) neutrophils

   C) antibodies

   D) natural killer lymphocytes

   C) is correct. Antibodies are part of the body's adaptive immune system and only respond to specific pathogens.

2. Which is NOT an external barrier to pathogens?

   A) earwax

   B) skin

   C) inflammation

   D) mucus

   C) is correct. Inflammation is a response to infection, not a barrier.

The Reproductive System

The Male Reproductive System

The male reproductive system produces SPERM, or male gametes, and passes them to the female reproductive system. Sperm are produced in the TESTES (also called testicles), which are housed externally in a sac-like structure called the SCROTUM. The scrotum contracts and relaxes to move the testes closer or farther from the body. This process keeps the testes at the appropriate temperature for sperm production, which is slightly lower than regular body temperature.

Mature sperm are stored in the EPIDIDYMIS. During sexual stimulation, sperm travel from the epididymis through a long, thin tube called the VAS DEFERENS. Along the way, the sperm is joined by fluids from three glands to form SEMEN. The SEMINAL VESICLES secrete the bulk of the fluid which makes up semen, which is composed of various proteins, sugars, and enzymes. The PROSTATE contributes an alkaline fluid that counteracts the acidity of the vaginal tract. Finally, the COWPER GLAND secretes a protein-rich fluid that acts as a lubricant. Semen travels through the URETHRA and exits the body through the PENIS, which becomes rigid during sexual arousal.

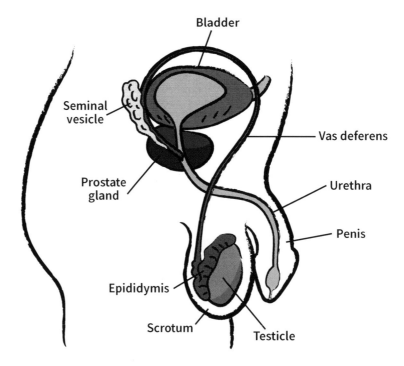

Figure 6.10. The Male Reproductive System

The main hormone associated with the male reproductive system is TESTOSTERONE, which is released by the testes (and in the adrenal glands in much smaller amounts). Testosterone is responsible for the development of the male reproductive system and male secondary sexual characteristics, including muscle development and facial hair growth.

The Female Reproductive System

The female reproductive system produces EGGS, or female gametes, and gestates the fetus during pregnancy. Eggs are produced in the OVARIES and travel through the FALLOPIAN TUBES to the UTERUS, which is a muscular organ that houses the fetus during pregnancy. The uterine cavity is lined with a layer of blood-rich tissue called the ENDOMETRIUM. If no pregnancy occurs, the endometrium is shed monthly during MENSTRUATION.

FERTILIZATION occurs when the egg absorbs the sperm; it usually takes place in the fallopian tubes but may happen in the uterus itself. After fertilization the new zygote implants itself in the endometrium, where it will grow and develop over thirty-eight weeks (roughly nine months). During gestation, the developing fetus acquires nutrients and passes waste through the PLACENTA.

This temporary organ is attached to the wall of the uterus and is connected to the baby by the UMBILICAL CORD.

When the fetus is mature, powerful muscle contractions occur in the myometrium, the muscular layer next to the endometrium. These contractions push the fetus through an opening called the CERVIX into the vagina, from which it exits the body. The placenta and umbilical cords are also expelled through the vagina shortly after birth.

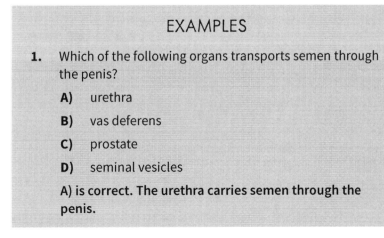

What type of muscle is most likely found in the myometrium of the uterus?

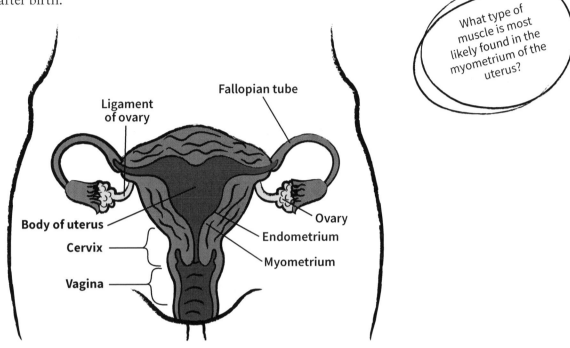

Figure 6.11. The Female Reproductive System

The female reproductive cycle is controlled by a number of different hormones. Estrogen, produced by the ovaries, stimulates Graafian follicles, which contain immature eggs cells. The pituitary gland then releases luteinizing hormone, which causes the egg to be released into the fallopian tubes during OVULATION. During pregnancy, estrogen and progesterone are released in high levels to help with fetal growth and to prevent further ovulation.

EXAMPLES

1. Which of the following organs transports semen through the penis?

   A) urethra

   B) vas deferens

   C) prostate

   D) seminal vesicles

   A) is correct. The urethra carries semen through the penis.

The Endocrine System

The endocrine system is composed of a network of organs called **GLANDS** that produce signaling chemicals called **HORMONES**. These hormones are released by glands into the bloodstream and then travel to the other tissues and organs whose functions they regulate. When they reach their target, hormones bond to a specific receptor on cell membranes, which affects the machinery of the cell. Hormones play an important role in regulating almost all bodily functions, including digestion, respiration, sleep, stress, growth, development, reproduction, and immune response.

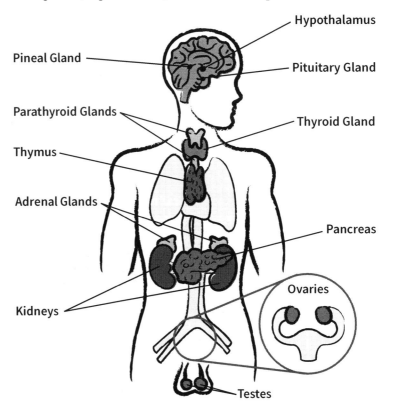

Figure 6.12. The Endocrine System

Much of the action of the endocrine system runs through the **HYPOTHALAMUS**, which is highly integrated into the nervous system. The hypothalamus receives signals from the brain and in turn will release hormones that regulate both other endocrine organs and important metabolic processes. Other endocrine glands include the pineal, pituitary, thyroid, parathyroid, thymus, and adrenal glands.

Organs from other systems, including the reproductive and digestive systems, can also secrete hormones, and thus are considered part of the endocrine system. The reproductive organs in both males (testes) and females (ovaries and placenta) release important hormones, as do the pancreas, liver, and stomach.

Table 6.2. Endocrine Glands

GLAND	REGULATES	HORMONES PRODUCED
pineal gland	circadian rhythms (the sleep/wake cycle)	melatonin
pituitary gland	growth, blood pressure, reabsorption of water by the kidneys, temperature, pain relief, and some reproductive functions related to pregnancy and childbirth	human growth hormone (HGH), thyroid-stimulating hormone (TSH), prolactin (PRL), luteinizing hormone (LH), follicle-stimulating hormone (FSH), oxytocin, antidiuretic hormone (ADH)
hypothalamus	pituitary function and metabolic processes including body temperature, hunger, thirst, and circadian rhythms	thyrotropin-releasing hormone (TRH), dopamine, growth-hormone-releasing hormone (GHRH), gonadotropin-releasing hormone (GnRH), oxytocin, vasopressin
thyroid gland	energy use and protein synthesis	thyroxine (T4), triiodothyronine (T3), calcitonin
parathyroid	calcium and phosphate levels	parathyroid hormone (PTH), calcitonin
adrenal glands	"fight or flight" response, regulation of salt and blood volume	epinephrine, norepinephrine, cortisol, androgens
pancreas	blood sugar levels and metabolism	insulin, glucagon, somatostatin
testes	maturation of sex organs, secondary sex characteristics	androgens (e.g., testosterone)
ovaries	maturation of sex organs, secondary sex characteristics, pregnancy, childbirth, and lactation	progesterone, estrogens
placenta	gestation and childbirth	progesterone, estrogens, human chorionic gonadotropin, human placental lactogen

Pathologies of the Endocrine System

Disruption of hormone production in specific endocrine glands can lead to disease. An inability to produce insulin results in uncontrolled blood glucose levels, a condition called DIABETES. Over- or underactive glands can lead to conditions like HYPOTHYROIDISM, which is characterized by slow metabolism, and hyperparathyroidism, which can lead to osteoporosis. Tumors on endocrine glands can also damage the functioning of a wide variety of bodily systems.

EXAMPLES

1. Which gland in the endocrine system is responsible for regulating blood glucose levels?

   A) adrenal

   B) testes

   C) pineal

   D) pancreas

   D) is correct. The pancreas releases insulin and glucagon, which regulate glucose levels in the blood.

2. Damage to the parathyroid would most likely affect which of the following?

   A) stress levels

   B) bone density

   C) secondary sex characteristics

   D) circadian rhythms

   B) is correct. The parathyroid controls calcium and phosphate levels, which are maintained by producing and reabsorbing bone tissue.

The Integumentary System

The INTEGUMENTARY SYSTEM refers to the skin (the largest organ in the body) and related structures, including the hair and nails. Skin is composed of three layers. The EPIDERMIS is the outermost layer of the skin. This waterproof layer contains no blood vessels and acts mainly to protect the body. Under the epidermis lies the DERMIS, which consists of dense connective tissue that allows skin to stretch and flex. The dermis is home to blood vessels, glands, and HAIR FOLLICLES. The HYPODERMIS is a layer of fat below the dermis that stores energy (in the form of fat) and acts as a cushion for the body. The hypodermis is sometimes called the SUBCUTANEOUS LAYER.

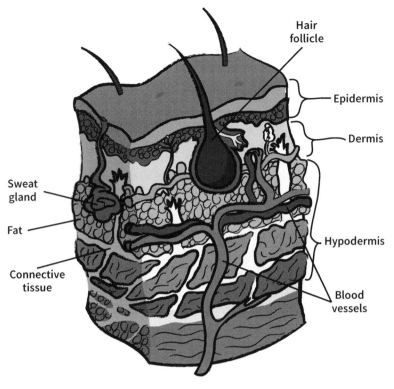

Figure 6.13. The Skin

The skin has several important roles. It acts as a barrier to protect the body from injury, the intrusion of foreign particles, and the loss of water and nutrients. It is also important for THERMOREGULA-TION. Blood vessels near the surface of the skin can dilate, allowing for higher blood flow and the release of heat. They can also constrict to reduce the amount of blood that travels near the surface of the skin, which helps conserve heat. The skin also produces vitamin D when exposed to sunlight.

Because the skin covers the whole body, it plays a vital role in allowing organisms to interact with the environment. It is home to nerve endings that sense temperature, pressure, and pain, and it also houses glands that help maintain homeostasis. ECCRINE glands, which are located primarily in the palms of the hands and soles of the feet (and to a lesser degree in other areas of the body), release the water and salt (NaCl) mixture called SWEAT. These glands help the body maintain the appropriate salt/water balance. Sweat can also contain small amounts of other substances the body needs to expel, including alcohol, lactic acid, and urea.

APOCRINE glands, which are located primarily in the armpit and groin, release an oily substance that contains pheromones. They are also sensitive to adrenaline, and are responsible for most of the sweating that occurs due to stress, fear, anxiety, or pain. Apocrine glands are largely inactive until puberty.

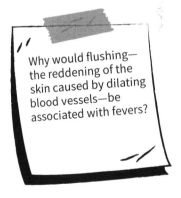

Why would flushing—the reddening of the skin caused by dilating blood vessels—be associated with fevers?

The Genitourinary System

The **URINARY SYSTEM** excretes water and waste from the body and is crucial for maintaining the body's electrolyte balance (the balance of water and salt in the blood). Because many organs function as part of both the reproductive and urinary systems, the two are sometimes referred to collectively as the **GENITOURINARY SYSTEM**.

The main organs of the urinary system are the **KIDNEYS**, which filter waste from the blood; maintain the electrolyte balance in the blood; and regulate blood volume, pressure, and pH. The kidneys also function as an endocrine organ and release several important hormones. These include **RENIN**, which regulates blood pressure, and **CALCITRIOL**, the active form of vitamin D. The kidney is divided into two regions: the **RENAL CORTEX**, which is the outermost layer, and the **RENAL MEDULLA**, which is the inner layer.

The functional unit of the kidney is the **NEPHRON**, which is a series of looping tubes that filter electrolytes, metabolic waste, and other water-soluble waste molecules from the blood. These wastes include **UREA**, which is a nitrogenous byproduct of protein catabolism, and **URIC ACID**, a byproduct of nucleic acid metabolism. Together, these waste products are excreted from the body in **URINE**.

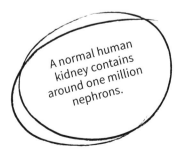

A normal human kidney contains around one million nephrons.

Filtration begins in a network of capillaries called a **GLOMERULUS** which is located in the renal cortex of each kidney. This waste is then funneled into **COLLECTING DUCTS** in the renal medulla.

From the collecting ducts, urine passes through the RENAL PELVIS and then through two long tubes called URETERS.

The two ureters drain into the urinary bladder, which holds up to 1000 milliliters of liquid. The bladder exit is controlled by two sphincters, both of which must open for urine to pass. The internal sphincter is made of smooth involuntary muscle, while the external sphincter can be voluntarily controlled. In males, the external sphincter also closes to prevent movement of seminal fluid into the bladder during sexual activity.

Urine exits the bladder through the URETHRA. In males, the urethra goes through the penis and also carries semen. In females, the much-shorter urethra ends just above the vaginal opening.

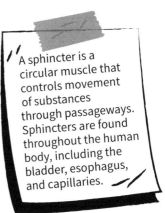

A sphincter is a circular muscle that controls movement of substances through passageways. Sphincters are found throughout the human body, including the bladder, esophagus, and capillaries.

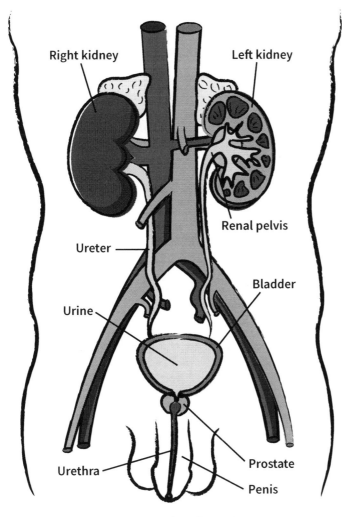

Figure 6.14. Genitourinary System

GO ON

EXAMPLES

1. Which of the following is the outermost layer of the kidney?

   A) renal cortex

   B) renal medulla

   C) renal pelvis

   D) nephron

   A) is correct. The outermost layer of the kidney is the renal cortex.

2. Which of the following organs holds urine before it passes into the urethra?

   A) prostate

   B) kidney

   C) ureter

   D) urinary bladder

   D) is correct. The urinary bladder holds urine before it passes to the urethra to be excreted.

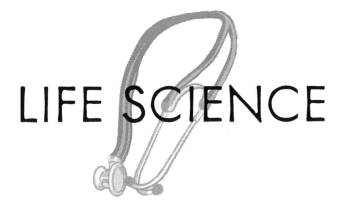

seven

LIFE SCIENCE

Biological Macromolecules

There are four basic biological macromolecules that are common between all organisms: carbohydrates, lipids, nucleic acids, and proteins. These molecules make life possible by performing basic cellular functions.

Macromolecules are **POLYMERS**, which are large molecules comprised of smaller molecules called **MONOMERS**. The monomers are joined together in an endothermic (energy requiring) dehydration reaction, so-called because it releases a molecule of water. Conversely, the bonds in polymers can be broken by an exothermic (energy-releasing) reaction that requires water.

Carbohydrates

CARBOHYDRATES, commonly known as sugars, are made up of carbon, hydrogen, and oxygen. The monomers of carbohydrates, called **MONOSACCHARIDES**, have these elements in the ratio $C_nH_{2n}O_n$. Common monosaccharides include glucose and fructose. These monomers join together to form **DISACCHARIDES**, such as sucrose and lactase, and **POLYSACCHARIDES**. These in turn can join together to form complex, branching molecules called **OLIGOSACCHARIDES**.

Carbohydrates are often taken into the body through ingestion of food and serve a number of purposes, acting as:

◆ fuel sources (glycogen, amylose)

◆ means of communication between cells (glycoproteins)

◆ cell structure support (cellulose, chitin)

Carbohydrates are broken down to their constituent parts for fuel and other biological functions. Inability to process sugars can lead to health issues; for example, inability to break down lactose (often due to problems with the enzyme LACTASE, which serves this function) leads to lactose intolerance, and problems with INSULIN not working properly in the breakdown of sugars can lead to DIABETES.

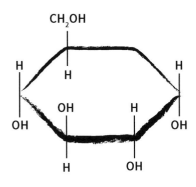

Figure 7.1. Glucose

Lipids

LIPIDS, commonly known as fats, are composed mainly of hydrogen and carbon. They serve a number of functions depending on their particular structure: they make up the outer structure of cells, and can act as fuel, as steroids, and as hormones. Lipids are hydrophobic, meaning they repel water.

Cholesterol is one example of a lipid, and is essential for normal functioning, although excessive accumulation can cause inflammation issues and high blood pressure. There are two types of cholesterol: HIGH-DENSITY LIPOPROTEIN (**HDL**) and LOW-DENSITY LIPOPROTEIN (**LDL**), with HDL commonly referred to as "good" cholesterol and LDL as "bad" cholesterol, as high levels of LDL in particular can cause health problems.

Proteins

PROTEINS serve an incredibly wide variety of purposes within the body. As enzymes, they play key roles in important processes like DNA replication, cellular division, and cellular metabolism. Structural proteins provide rigidity to cartilage, hair, nails, and the cytoskeletons (the network of molecules that hold the parts of a cell in place). They are also involved in communication between cells and in the transportation of molecules.

Proteins are composed of individual AMINO ACIDS, each of which has an amino group and carboxylic acid group, along with other side groups. Amino acids are joined together by PEPTIDE BONDS to form polypeptides. There are twenty amino acids, and the order of the amino acids in the polypeptide determines the shape and function of the molecule.

Nucleic Acids

NUCLEIC ACIDS store hereditary information and are composed of monomers called **NUCLEOTIDES**. Each nucleotide includes a sugar, a phosphate group, and a nitrogenous base.

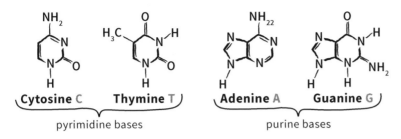

Figure 7.2. Nucleotides

There are two types of nucleic acids. **DEOXYRIBONUCLEIC ACID** (**DNA**) contains the genetic instructions to produce proteins. It is composed of two strings of nucleotides wound into a double helix shape. The backbone of the helix is made from the nucleotide's sugar (deoxyribose) and phosphate groups. The "rungs" of the ladder are made from one of four nitrogenous bases: adenine, thymine, cytosine, and guanine. These bases bond together in specific pairs: adenine with thymine and cytosine with guanine.

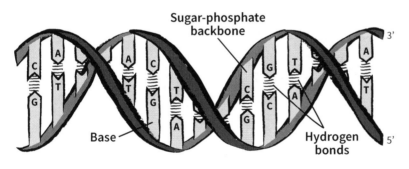

Figure 7.3. DNA

RIBONUCLEIC ACID (**RNA**) transcribes information from DNA and plays several vital roles in the replication of DNA and the manufacturing of proteins. RNA nucleotides contain a sugar (ribose), a phosphate group, and one of four nitrogenous bases: adenine, uracil, cytosine, and guanine. It is usually found as a single stranded molecule.

The Structure and Role of DNA

DNA stores information by coding for proteins using blocks of three nucleotides called **CODONS**. Each codon codes for a specific amino acid; together, all the codons needed to make a specific

There are three main differences between DNA and RNA:

1. DNA contains the nucleotide thymine; RNA contains the nucleotide uracil.
2. DNA is double stranded; RNA is single stranded.
3. DNA is made from the sugar deoxyribose; RNA is made from the sugar ribose.

protein are called a GENE. In addition to codons for specific amino acids, there are also codons that signal "start" and "stop."

When a protein is produced, the two sides of the DNA helix unwind, and a complementary strand of messenger RNA (mRNA) is manufactured using the DNA as a template (a process called transcription). This mRNA then travels outside the nucleus where it is "read" by a ribosome (a process called translation). Each codon is matched to an ANTI-CODON, which carries a specific amino acid. The sequence of amino acids is then joined together to form a polypeptide.

A MUTATION causes a change in the sequence of nucleotides within DNA. For example, the codon GAC codes for the amino acid aspartic acid. However, if the cytosine is swapped for an adenine, the codon now reads GAA, which corresponds to the amino acid glutamic acid.

When it is not being transcribed, DNA is tightly wound around proteins called HISTONES into packages called CHROMATIN. The structure of chromatin allows large amounts of DNA to be stored in a very small space and helps regulate transcription by controlling access to specific sections of DNA. Tightly folding the DNA also helps prevent damage to the genetic code. Chromatin is further bundled into packages of DNA called CHROMOSOMES. During cell division, DNA is replicated to create two identical copies of each chromosome called CHROMATIDS.

How might a mutation in a single codon affect the finished protein?

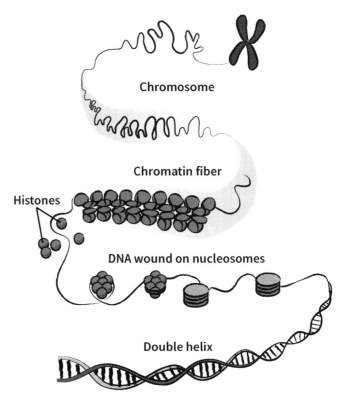

Chromosome

Chromatin fiber

Histones

DNA wound on nucleosomes

Double helix

Figure 7.4. DNA, Chromatin, and Chromosomes

1. Which of the following is NOT an amino acid found in DNA?

   A) adenine

   B) guanine

   C) uracil

   D) thymine

   C) is correct. Uracil is found only in RNA.

2. Which of the following processes uses the information stored in RNA to produce a protein?

   A) replication

   B) translation

   C) transcription

   D) mutation

   B) is correct. Translation is the process of matching codons in RNA to the correct anti-codon to manufacture a protein.

3. Which of the following is a monomer used to build carbohydrates?

   A) glucose

   B) thymine

   C) aspartic acid

   D) histone

   A) is correct. Glucose is a monosaccharide that can be used to build larger polysaccharides.

The Cell

A CELL is the smallest unit of life that can reproduce on its own. Unicellular organisms, such as amoebae, are made up of only one cell, while multicellular organisms are comprised of many cells. Cells consist of many different parts that work together to maintain the life of the cell.

Cell Membranes

The outer surface of human cells is made up of a PLASMA MEMBRANE, which gives the cell its shape. This membrane is primarily composed of a PHOSPHOLIPID BILAYER, which itself is made up of two layers of lipids facing in opposing directions. This functions to separate the inner cellular environment from the EXTRACELLULAR SPACE, the space between cells. CHANNEL PROTEINS, embedded in the phospholipid bilayer, allow specialized molecular transport into and out of the cell. In addition, through a process known as OSMOSIS, in which certain particles can pass through a membrane, molecules can pass into or out of the cell at the plasma membrane as needed.

Cell Organelles

Within the cell, specialized parts known as ORGANELLES serve individual functions to support the cell. The inside of the cell (excluding the nucleus) is the CYTOPLASM, which includes both organelles and CYTOSOL, a fluid that aids in molecular transport and reactions.

The function of individual organelles can be compared to the functions of components in a city. The "power plant" for the cell is its mitochondria, which produce energy for the cell in the form of ADENOSINE TRIPHOSPHATE (ATP). This process is known as CELLULAR RESPIRATION, as it requires oxygen that is taken in from the lungs and supplied in blood. Byproducts of cellular respiration are water and carbon dioxide, the latter of which is transported into blood and then to the lungs, where it is exhaled.

The "city hall" of the cell is the cell NUCLEUS, which is where the cell's "instructions" governing its functions originate. The nucleus contains the cell's DNA and is surrounded by a NUCLEAR MEMBRANE. Only eukaryotic cells have nuclei; prokaryotic nucleic acids are not contained with a membrane-bound organelle.

The transporting "railway" function is largely served by ENDO-PLASMIC RETICULUM. Proteins and lipids travel along endoplasmic reticulum as they are constructed and transported within the cell. There are two types of endoplasmic reticulum, SMOOTH and ROUGH, which are distinguished by the fact that the latter is embedded with RIBOSOMES. Also, smooth endoplasmic reticulum are associated with the production and transport of lipids, whereas rough endoplasmic reticulum are associated with the production and transport of proteins. Ribosomes themselves are sites of protein production; here, molecules produced from the nucleus-encoding proteins guide the assembly of proteins from amino acids.

Similarly, the GOLGI APPARATUS is another organelle involved in protein synthesis and transport. After a new protein is synthesized at the ribosome and travels along the endoplasmic reticulum, the Golgi apparatus packages it into a VESICLE (essentially a plasma membrane "bubble"), which can then be transported within the cell or secreted outside of the cell, as needed.

Plant cells include a number of structures not found in animal cells. These include the CELL WALL, which provides the cell with a hard outer structure, and chloroplasts, where PHOTOSYNTHESIS occurs. During photosynthesis, plants store energy from sunlight as sugars, which serve as the main source of energy for cell functions.

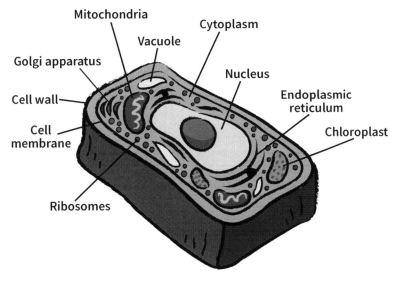

Figure 7.5. Plant Cell

The Cell Cycle

From the very earliest moments of life throughout adulthood, cell division is a critical function of cell biology. The rate of division differs between cell types; hair and skin cells divide relatively rapidly (which is why chemotherapy drugs, which target rapidly-dividing cells in an effort to destroy cancerous cells, often cause hair loss), whereas liver cells rarely divide, except in response to injury. Regardless of cell type (with the exception of reproductive cells), the process of cell division follows consistent stages, which make up the CELL CYCLE.

The cell cycle is made up of five stages. Cells at rest, which are not dividing, are considered to be at the G_0 (GROWTH PHASE 0) stage of the cell cycle. Once cell division is triggered (for example, by extracellular signals in response to nearby damage, requiring new cells to replace the damaged cells), cells enter stage G_1. In this stage, the organelles of the soon-to-be-dividing cell are duplicated, in order to support both daughter cells upon division. Similarly, in the next stage, **S (DNA SYNTHESIS) PHASE**, the genetic material of the cell (DNA) is duplicated, to ensure that each cell has the full complement of genetic instructions. Additional growth and protein production occurs in the subsequent stage, G_2 PHASE.

G_1, S, and G_2 are collectively known as INTERPHASE, in which the cell is growing and preparing to divide; the subsequent stages in which the cell is actively dividing are stages of MITOSIS. The first mitotic stage is PROPHASE, in which the newly replicated DNA condenses into chromosomes. These chromosomes are in pairs (humans have twenty-three pairs of chromosomes), with each pair joined together at the CENTROMERE.

Next, in PROMETAPHASE, the nuclear membrane breaks down. KINETOCHORES form on chromosomes, which are proteins that attach to kinetochore MICROTUBULES (cellular filaments) anchored at opposite ends of the cell. In METAPHASE, the chromosomes align along the center of the cell, perpendicular to the poles anchoring the microtubules. The alignment is such that one of each chromosome duplicates is attached to each pole by these microtubules.

In ANAPHASE, the microtubules pull the duplicates apart from each other toward each of the poles. In the final mitosis stage, TELOPHASE, nuclei reform in each pole of the cell, and cellular filaments contract to divide the cell into two cells, both with a full complement of genetic material and organelles. Following mitosis, both daughter cells return to the G_1 phase, either to begin the process of division once again or to rest without dividing (G_0).

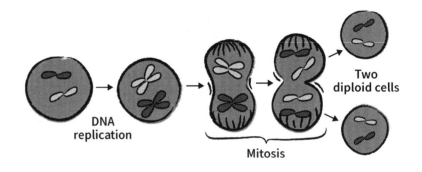

Figure 7.6. Mitosis

The process of producing sex cells (GAMETES: OVUM for women and SPERMATOZOA for men) is similar to mitosis, except that it produces cells with only half the normal number of chromosomes. Thus, when two sex cells fuse, the resulting ZYGOTE has the proper amount of chromosomes (and genetic information from both parents). This process is known as MEIOSIS.

In the prophase of meiosis, chromosome pairs align next to each other. At this stage, transfer of genetic material can occur between members of each pair, in a process known as HOMOLOGOUS RECOMBINATION, which can increase the genetic diversity of offspring.

In meiotic metaphase, these chromosomes align as pairs in the center of the cell, and the chromosomes are separated during anaphase. As a result, each gamete cell ends up with one copy of each chromosome pair, and thus one half of the genetic complement necessary for the zygote.

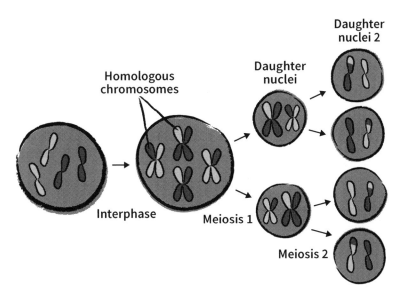

Figure 7.7. Meiosis

EXAMPLES

1. Cellular respiration produces which of the following molecules?

   A) oxygen

   B) ADP

   C) ATP

   D) glucose

   C) is correct. Oxygen and glucose are used, not produced, in this process. ADP is used to produce ATP.

2. Which of the following houses the cell's DNA?

   A) rough endoplasmic reticulum

   B) smooth endoplasmic reticulum

   C) mitochondrion

   D) nucleus

   D) is correct. Smooth and rough endoplasmic reticula process and transport lipids and proteins, and mitochondria produce the cell's chemical energy.

3. Which of the following processes creates daughter cells with half the number of chromosomes contained in somatic (body) cells?

   A) mitosis

   B) meiosis

   C) recombination

   D) the cell cycle

B) is correct. Meiosis produces sex cells, which have half the number of chromosomes that somatic cells contain. Mitosis produces somatic cells, and recombination refers to the movement of DNA between chromosomes. The cell cycle includes the entire lifecycle of a cell, which may include mitosis or meiosis.

Genetics

Heredity

When organisms reproduce, GENETIC information is passed to the next generation through DNA. Within DNA are blocks of nucleotides called genes, each of which contains the code needed to produce a specific protein. Genes are responsible for TRAITS, or characteristics, in organisms such as eye color, height, and flower color. The sequence of nucleotides in DNA is called an organism's GENOTYPE, while the resulting physical traits are the organism's PHENOTYPE.

Different versions of the same gene (e.g., one that codes for blue eyes and one for green eyes) are called ALLELES. During sexual reproduction, the child receives two alleles of each gene—one each on the mother's chromosomes and the father's chromosomes. These alleles can be HOMOZYGOUS (identical) or HETEROZYGOUS (different). If the organism is heterozygous for a particular gene, which allele is expressed is determined by which alleles are dominant and/or recessive. According to the rules of Mendelian heredity, DOMINANT alleles will always be expressed, while RECESSIVE alleles are only expressed if the organism has no dominant alleles for that gene.

The genotype, and resulting phenotype, of sexually reproducing organisms can be tracked using Punnett squares, which show the alleles of the PARENT GENERATION on each of two axes. (Note that dominant alleles are always depicted using capital letters while recessive alleles are written in lower case.) The possible phenotype of the resulting offspring, called the **F1** GENERATION, are then shown in the body of the square. The squares do not show the phenotype of any one offspring; instead, they show the ratio of phenotypes found across the generation. In Figure 7.8, two heterozygous parents for trait *R* are mated, resulting in a ratio of 1:2:1 for homozygous dominant, heterozygous, and homozygous recessive. Note that this creates a 3:1 ratio of dominant to recessive phenotypes.

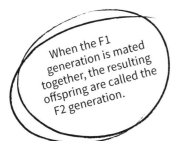

Many of the rules of genetics were discovered by Gregor Mendel, a nineteenth century abbot who used pea plants to show how traits are passed down through generations.

When the F1 generation is mated together, the resulting offspring are called the F2 generation.

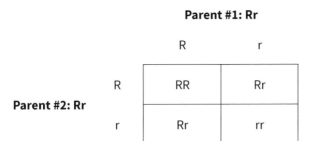

Figure 7.8. Punnett Square

Similarly, crossing two parents that are heterozygous for two traits (dihybrids) results in a phenotypic ratio of 9:3:3:1, as shown below. This ratio is known as the DIHYBRID RATIO.

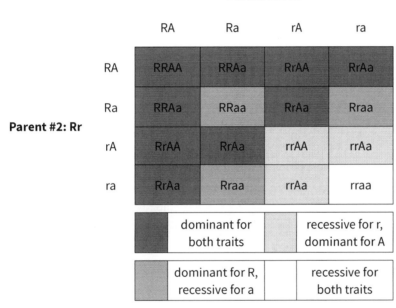

Figure 7.9. Dihybrid Cross

Non-Mendelian inheritance describes patterns in inheritance that do not follow the ratios described above. The patterns can occur for a number of reasons. Alleles might show incomplete dominance, meaning multiple alleles will be expressed. Thus, the resulting phenotype might include several distinct traits (such as the AB blood type) or be a mix of two traits (for example, a red flower and white flower cross to create a pink flower). The expression of genes can also be regulated by mechanisms other than the dominant/recessive relationship. For example, some genes may inhibit the expression of other genes, a process called epistasis. The environment can also impact gene expression. For example, organisms with the same genotype may grow to different sizes depending on the nutrients available to them.

When a person's genetic code is damaged, that organism may have a GENETIC DISORDER. For example, cystic fibrosis, which causes difficulty with basic bodily functions such as breathing and eating, results from damage to the gene which codes for a protein called CFTR. Down syndrome, which causes developmental delays, occurs when a person has three copies of chromosome 21 (meaning they received two copies from a parent as a result of an error in meiosis).

Natural Selection and Evolution

Genes are not static. Over time, MUTATIONS, or changes in the genetic code, occur that can affect an organism's ability to survive. Harmful mutations will appear less often in a population or be removed entirely because those organisms will be less likely to reproduce (and thus will not pass on that trait). Beneficial mutations may help an organism reproduce, and thus that trait will appear more often. Over time, this process, called NATURAL SELECTION, results in the evolution of new species. The theory of evolution was developed by naturalist Charles Darwin when he observed how finches on the Galapagos Islands had a variety of beak shapes and sizes that allowed them to coexist by using different food sources.

As a result of these processes, all organisms share a distant evolutionary predecessor. As evolution progressed, species subsequently split off as different branches of the phylogenetic (evolutionary) tree of species diversity, leading to the complexity of life seen today. For example, humans share a recent evolutionary ancestor with other primates (but did not evolve directly from any of these species).

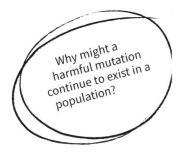

Why might a harmful mutation continue to exist in a population?

EXAMPLES

1. If a plant that is homozygous dominant (**T**) for a trait is crossed with a plant that is homozygous recessive (**t**) for the same trait, what will be the phenotype of the offspring if the trait follows Mendelian patterns of inheritance?

    A) All offspring will show the dominant phenotype.

    B) All offspring will show the recessive phenotype.

    C) Half the offspring will show the dominant trait, and the other half will show the recessive phenotype.

    D) All the offspring will show a mix of the dominant and recessive phenotypes.

    A) is correct. Because each offspring will inherit the dominant allele, all the offspring will show the dominant phenotype. The offspring would only show a mix of the two phenotypes if they did not follow Mendelian inheritance patterns.

2. Which of the following mutations would most likely be passed on to an organism's offspring?

A) a mutation that prevents the production of functioning sperm cells

B) a mutation that causes the deterioration of nerve cells in mature adults

C) a mutation that does not cause any changes to the organism's phenotype

D) a mutation that limits the growth of bone cells in children

B) is correct. Because this mutation presents in older adults who have likely already reproduced, it is likely to have been passed on to the next generation. Mutations that affect reproduction and children are much less likely to be passed on. A mutation that causes no changes in phenotype may either disappear or spread as a result of random fluctuations in the gene pool.

eight

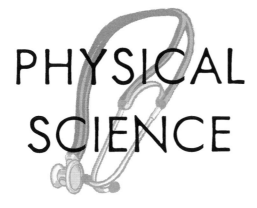

PHYSICAL SCIENCE

Properties of Atoms

An ATOM is defined as the smallest constituent unit of an element that still retains all of the original properties of the element, and all matter is composed of atoms. Atoms are not irreducible, however, and may be broken into further components: protons, neutrons, and electrons. All atomic nuclei are comprised of positively charged protons and neutrally charged neutrons, such that nuclei have an overall positive charge. Negatively charged electrons orbit the nucleus at various energy levels. Thus, overall atomic charge is determined by the number of positively charged protons and negatively charged electrons in an atom.

The attraction between the opposite charges of the protons and electrons is responsible for holding an atom together. Nuclear forces, or the attraction between protons and neutrons, hold nuclei together, meaning that they are stronger than electrical forces that would otherwise break an atom apart.

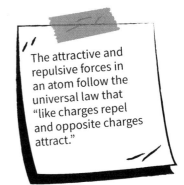

The attractive and repulsive forces in an atom follow the universal law that "like charges repel and opposite charges attract."

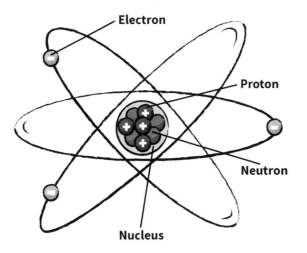

Figure 8.1. Structure of an Atom

Each element has a distinctive number of protons; this number defines the identity of the atom. The order of elements on the Periodic Table from top to bottom and left to right indicates their number of protons; that number is an element's ATOMIC NUMBER. Hydrogen, the first element on the periodic table, has one proton while helium, the second element, has two, and so on.

Along with atomic charge, atoms have measurable mass. Protons and neutrons are significantly more massive than electrons (about 1,800 times), so the mass of electrons is not considered when calculating the mass of an atom. Thus, an element's MASS NUMBER is the number of protons and neutrons present in its atoms.

While atoms of the same element have the same number of protons, their number of neutrons may vary. Atoms which differ in their number of neutrons but have equal numbers of protons are ISOTOPES of the same element. Some isotopes are radioactive, which means that they spontaneously undergo nuclear reactions and decay (release subatomic particles). Because the rate of decay for each isotope is generally predictable, this decay may be used to estimate the age of radioactive materials.

When writing the atomic symbol of an element, isotopes are differentiated by writing the number of neutrons in the upper right-hand corner of the symbol. One would write the atomic symbol for ordinary hydrogen as ^1H, to signify that it has only 1 neutron. While this is usually not done for the most common isotope of an element, it is necessary to distinguish its isotopes, such as deuterium and tritium, as ^2H and ^3H, respectively.

The ATOMIC MASS of an atom, which is different from the mass number, is the average mass of all known isotopes of an element. Thus, to determine the number of neutrons in a given atom, simply subtract the number of protons from the element's atomic mass. For each element on the Periodic Table, the atomic number is listed above the symbol of the element (for example, He for helium) and the atomic mass (measured in atomic mass units, or AMU) is listed underneath the symbol.

Atoms may lose or gain electrons during chemical reactions resulting in a charged atom, known as an ION. Ions are called CATIONS if they are positively charged due to the loss of electrons or ANIONS if they are negatively charged due to the gaining of electrons. Ionic charges are denoted by adding a plus or minus sign onto the elemental symbol; for example, a sodium ion with a charge of +1 would be written as Na+.

Ions may be composed of two or more atoms known as molecular ions or POLYATOMIC IONS. The overall charge of a polyatomic ion is equal to the sum of the charges of all constituent atoms.

atomic number = number of protons

mass number = number of protons + number of neutrons

atomic mass = average mass of all isotopes

Table 8.1. Polyatomic Ions

NH^{4+}	ammonium
H_3O^+	hydronium
PO_4^{3-}	phosphate
SO_4^{2-}	sulfate
MnO_4^{2-}	manganate
OH^-	hydroxide
CN^-	cyanide
CO_3^{2-}	carbonate
HCO_3^{2-}	hydrogen carbonate
ClO^{2-}	chlorite

The Periodic Table of the Elements

There are many useful physical and chemical patterns represented in the Periodic Table of the Elements. The periodic table is organized into rows called **PERIODS** and columns called **GROUPS**. The position of an element's symbol on the periodic table indicates its electron configuration. There are seven periods on the table, numbered from top to bottom, and the number of the period indicates the energy level of the highest-energy-filled orbital in an atom. The elements in each group on the table all contain the same amount of electrons in their valence shell, which results in all elements in a group having similar chemical properties.

1 H 1.0079																		2 He 4.0026
3 Li 6.9411	4 Be 9.0122												5 B 10.811	6 C 12.011	7 N 14.007	8 O 15.999	9 F 18.998	10 Ne 20.180
11 Na 22.990	12 Mg 24.305												13 Al 26.982	14 Si 28.086	15 P 30.974	16 S 32.065	17 Cl 35.453	18 Ar 39.948
19 K 39.098	20 Ca 40.078		21 Sc 44.956	22 Ti 47.867	23 V 50.942	24 Cr 51.996	25 Mn 54.938	26 Fe 55.845	27 Co 58.933	28 Ni 58.693	29 Cu 63.546	30 Zn 65.39	31 Ga 69.723	32 Ge 72.61	33 As 74.922	34 Se 78.96	35 Br 79.904	36 Kr 83.80
37 Rb 85.468	38 Sr 87.62		39 Y 88.906	40 Zr 91.224	41 Nb 92.906	42 Mo 95.94	43 Tc [98]	44 Ru 101.07	45 Rh 102.91	46 Pd 106.42	47 Ag 107.87	48 Cd 112.41	49 In 114.82	50 Sn 118.71	51 Sb 121.76	52 Te 127.60	53 I 126.90	54 Xe 131.29
55 Cs 132.91	56 Ba 137.33	57-70 *	71 Lu 174.97	72 Hf 178.49	73 Ta 180.95	74 W 183.84	75 Re 186.21	76 Os 190.23	77 Ir 192.22	78 Pt 195.08	79 Au 196.97	80 Hg 200.59	81 Tl 204.38	82 Pb 207.2	83 Bi 208.98	84 Po [209]	85 At [210]	86 Rn [222]
87 Fr [223]	88 Ra [226]	89-102 * *	103 Lr [262]	104 Rf [261]	105 Db [262]	106 Sg [266]	107 Bh [264]	108 Hs [269]	109 Mt [268]	110 Uun [271]	111 Uuu [272]	112 Uub [277]		114 Uuq [289]				

* Lanthanide Series	57 La 138.91	58 Ce 140.12	59 Pr 140.91	60 Nd 144.24	61 Pm [145]	62 Sm 150.36	63 Eu 151.96	64 Gd 157.25	65 Tb 158.93	66 Dy 162.50	67 Ho 164.93	68 Er 167.26	69 Tm 168.93	70 Yb 173.04
* * Actinide Series	89 Ac [227]	90 Th 232.04	91 Pa 231.04	92 U 238.03	93 Np [237]	94 Pu [244]	95 Am [243]	96 Cm [247]	97 Bk [247]	98 Cf [251]	99 Es [252]	100 Fm [257]	101 Md [258]	102 No [259]

Figure 8.2. The Periodic Table of the Elements

Specific names are given to certain groups on the periodic table. Group 1 elements (belonging to the leftmost column) are known as the ALKALI METALS and are characterized by the fact that they are very unstable and react violently with water. Other notably reactive elements lie in Group 17, called the HALOGENS. In contrast with both of these groups, Group 18 contains the NOBLE GASES, which are inert and very non-reactive because they have a full outer shell of electrons.

There are two periods below and separated from the main periodic table. These are called LANTHANIDES and ACTINIDES. They are set apart from the other elements for two reasons: first, to consolidate the periodic table, and second, because they are more complicated chemically than the rest of the elements—which means that they do not follow any of the trends outlined below.

Keeping these exceptions in mind, trends for the remainder of the periodic table include the following, listed alphabetically:

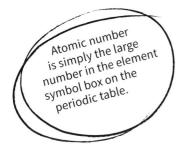

Atomic number is simply the large number in the element symbol box on the periodic table.

ATOMIC NUMBER: The atomic number (equal to the number of protons) of an element increases from left to right and top to bottom on the Periodic Table of the Elements. This means that hydrogen, with the lowest atomic number, is located at the upper left corner of the table.

ATOMIC RADIUS: Atomic radius increases from right to left and top to bottom on the periodic table, with the largest elements residing in the lower left corner.

ELECTRON AFFINITY: An atom's electron affinity refers to its ability to accept an electron. Electron affinity is measured quantitatively, using the amount of energy change that occurs when an electron is added to a neutral atom in its gaseous state. On the periodic table, electron affinity increases from left to right and bottom to top, with the highest electron affinities belonging to elements residing in the upper right corner.

ELECTRONEGATIVITY: Electronegativity measures how easily an atom can attract electrons and form chemical bonds. In general, electronegativity increases from left to right and bottom to top on the Periodic Table of the Elements, with fluorine being the most electronegative element. Electronegativity decreases from top to bottom of a group on the periodic table because of the increasing atomic radius, which corresponds with a greater distance between the electron orbital shells. One notable exception to these electronegativity trends is Group

QUICK REVIEW
Identify the least electronegative atom on the periodic table. Next, identify the most electronegative element on the table. Now draw a straight arrow from the least to the most electronegative element. This is the general trend of electronegativity.

18, the noble gases, since they possess a complete valence shell in their ground state and generally do not attract electrons.

Ionization Energy: The ionization energy of an element is defined as the energy necessary to remove an electron from a neutral atom in its gaseous phase. In other words, the lower this energy is, the more likely an atom is to lose an electron and become a cation. Ionization energies increase from left to right and bottom to top on the periodic table, meaning that the lowest ionization energies are in the lower left corner and the highest are in the upper right corner. This is because elements to the right on the periodic table are unlikely to lose electrons and become cations since their outer valence shells are nearly full.

Melting Point: An element's melting point is defined as the amount of energy that is required to change the substance from a solid phase to a liquid. This phase transition requires overcoming attractions between the molecules or atoms which comprise the substance. While melting points do not follow quite as straightforward a trend as many other characteristics, there are some observations that can be made with regard to the periodic table. Generally, most metals have a high melting point and non-metals have a low melting point. Carbon has the highest boiling point of the elements, with boron taking second place.

Metallic Character: The division between metals and non-metals on the table is a line that looks like a staircase, separating boron (B) from aluminum (Al), silicon (Si) from germanium (Ge), and so on all the way down to polonium (Po) which is separated from tellurium (Te) and astatine (At). Metallic properties increase from top to bottom and right to left on the Periodic Table, with the non-metals in the upper right corner and the most metallic elements in the lower left.

There are other important patterns to note as well. Elements on the left side of the periodic table are more likely to become cations, while elements on the right are more likely to become anions. This means that the left side of the periodic table has a positive valence while the right side has a negative one.

Recognize that electronegativity and ionization energy follow the same periodic trends. These two properties are simply different manifestations of the same atomic property: the strength with which an atom holds electrons.

Electron Configuration

Conventionally, electrons are depicted as orbiting a nucleus in defined pathways, much like a planet orbits the sun. In reality, electrons exist in clouds surrounding the atomic nucleus. These clouds are considered to be the orbital pathways and are defined as the volume of space in which an electron is 95 percent likely to be found.

A description of the locations of electrons in an atom is known as the atom's ELECTRON CONFIGURATION. An atom's electron configuration influences some of its physical and chemical properties, including boiling point, conductivity, and its propensity to engage in chemical reactions (also called the atom's stability). The chemical reactivity of an atom is determined by the electrons in the outermost shell, as they are first to interact with neighboring atoms.

These outermost electrons determine an atom's VALENCE number, which is the number of electrons that an atom will lose, gain, or share when it forms a compound. This number is usually equal to the number of electrons needed to fill the outermost orbital shell of an atom, which is known as the VALENCE SHELL. Most elements require eight electrons to fill their outermost shell. So, elements with six or seven valence electrons are likely to gain electrons (and become cations). Conversely, elements with one or two electrons are very likely to lose electrons (and become anions). Elements with exactly eight electrons (the noble gases), are almost completely unreactive.

There are four types of SUBSHELLS used to characterize an atom's electron configuration, labeled using the letters s, p, d, and f. Each letter label has a corresponding orbital shape within the subshells. For example, the s subshell is spherical, while the p subshell is shaped like a bow tie.

Each subshell contains a specific number of orbitals, and each orbital can hold two electrons. The 2 electrons are said to have opposite spins. The s subshell has 1 orbital, meaning it holds 2 electrons. The p subshell has 3 orbitals, meaning that it can hold up to 6 electrons. The d subshell has 5 orbitals and can hold up to 10 electrons, and the f subshell has 7 orbitals which can hold up to 14 electrons. The number of the orbital is denoted by an integer, and the number of electrons in that orbital is given as a superscript. For example, when the second p subshell is full, it is denoted as $2p^6$.

Electrons fill orbitals in a specific order that minimizes an atom's energy. Thus, the levels are filled in order of increasing energy as they are further and further from the atom's nucleus. In addition, according to HUND'S RULE, all empty orbitals are singly filled before electrons are paired. For example, the 3s shell contains 3 orbitals;

if it contains 4 electrons, it will have 1 orbital with 2 electrons, and 2 orbitals with 1 electron each (NOT 2 orbitals with 2 electrons each).

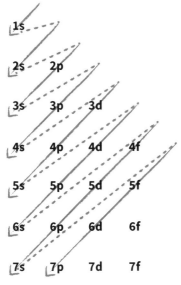

$$1s^2 2s^2 2p^6 3s^2 3p^6 4s^2 3d^{10} 4p^6 5s^2 ...$$

Figure 8.3. Electron Configuration

The electron configuration of each element correlates to its position on the periodic table: Group 1 and Group 2 (defined as the **S-BLOCK**) have valence electrons in s-orbitals. Alkali metals and helium (defined as the **P-BLOCK**) have valence electrons in their p-orbitals. Group 8 through Group 13 elements (defined as the **D-BLOCK**) have valence electrons in d-orbitals. Group 3 through Group 12 are a specific subset of d-block elements, defined as transition metals. The **F-BLOCK** is defined as elements with valence electrons in their f-orbitals and includes the two rows of lanthanides and actinides at the bottom of the periodic table, separated from the rest of the table.

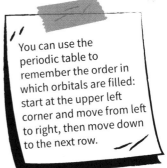

You can use the periodic table to remember the order in which orbitals are filled: start at the upper left corner and move from left to right, then move down to the next row.

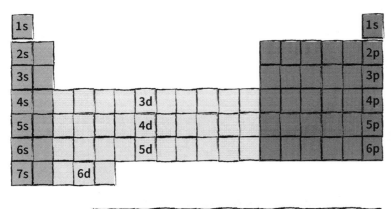

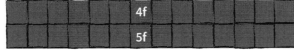

Figure 8.4. Electron Orbitals on the Periodic Table

Instead of tediously writing the entire electron configuration for an element, scientists abbreviate the notation of electron configurations. Consider the element Be, or beryllium. Its configuration is $1s^22s^2$, but can be simplified by writing $[He]2s^2$. This means that it has the electron configuration of helium, plus 2 additional electrons in the 2s subshell.

EXAMPLES

1. Rank the following in order of increasing atomic radius: xenon (Xe), barium (Ba), cesium (Cs).

   A) Xe < Cs < Ba

   B) Cs < Xe < Ba

   C) Ba < Cs < Xe

   D) Xe < Ba < Cs

   D) is correct. Atomic radius increases from the top of the periodic table to the bottom and also increases from right to left on the table. This means that the largest atoms are found in the lower-right-hand corner of the periodic table while the smallest are found in the upper-right-hand corner. Keeping this in mind, of the three elements listed, xenon has the smallest radius, barium is larger as it is further down and much further to the right, and cesium is the largest as it is furthest to the right of the three: Xe < Ba < Cs.

2. What is the electron configuration of ground-state neutral magnesium (Mg)?

   A) $1s^22s^22p^63s^2$

   B) $1s^22s^22p^23s^2$

   C) $1s^22s^62p^23s^2$

   D) $1s^22s^22p^23s^3$

   A) is correct. Mg has an atomic number of 12 on the periodic table. This means that ground-state neutral Mg has 12 protons and 12 electrons. These 12 electrons are assigned to orbitals in the order represented by the arrangement of the s-block and p-block on the periodic table: $1s^22s^22p^63s^2$.

3. List the following in order of decreasing electronegativity: fluorine (F), bromine (Br), magnesium (Mg), strontium (Sr).

   A) F > Mg > Br < Sr

   B) F > Br > Mg > Sr

   C) Br > Mg > Sr > F

   D) Sr > Mg > Br > F

   B) is correct. Electronegativity generally increases from bottom to top and from right to left on

Intramolecular Bonds

Chemical bonds, also called intramolecular bonds, are attractions between atoms that allow for the creation of substances consisting of more than one atom. When all the chemically bonded atoms are the same element, the substance is known as a MOLECULE. When two or more different elements bond together, the result is called a COMPOUND. (However, the word *molecule* is often used colloquially to refer to both types of substances.)

Table 8.2. Common Molecules and Compounds

H_2O	water
NaCl	table salt
CO_2	carbon dioxide
HCl	hydrochloric acid
O_3	ozone
$C_6H_{12}O_6$	glucose (sugar)
H_2	hydrogen gas

Not all chemical bonds are alike. Their causes vary, and thus the strength of those bonds also varies widely. There are two major types of bonds, distinguished from one another based on whether electrons are shared or transferred between the atoms. The first type of bond is a COVALENT BOND, which involves a pair of atoms sharing electrons from their outer s- and p-orbitals to fill their valence shell. Atoms bond covalently in order to gain the stability brought about by a full valence electron shell, but whether two atoms can bond depends on their electronegativity. Covalent bonds are generally formed between two non-metals with similar electronegativities.

The second type of bond is an IONIC BOND, which results from the attraction between ions. Ionic bonds occur between atoms with very different electronegativities; instead of sharing electrons, one atom "gives" its electrons to the other, resulting in one positively and one negatively charged atom.

Ionic bonds are weaker than covalent bonds since the ions are more easily susceptible to outside forces and attractions. Consider the example of sodium chloride, NaCl, which is ordinary table salt. While the bond in sodium chloride may seem strong given that table salt is solid at room temperature, this ionic bond will break immediately if sodium chloride is placed in water. It breaks apart because of the attractive forces of the water molecules, leaving separate Na^+ and Cl^- ions floating in the water. This observation can be generalized to all ionic compounds, which readily dissolve in water.

Besides electronegativity and strength, there are a few other important differences between covalent and ionic bonds. Covalently bonded compounds exist in liquid or gaseous phase at room temperature, while ionic compounds are solid. Also, covalent bonds have a definite geometry (or shape) while ionic bonds do not. Ionic bonds have a higher melting point and boiling point than covalent bonds.

A third type of bond, a METALLIC BOND, also results from the sharing of electrons, but instead of sharing electrons in a specific valence shell, metallic bonds are generally described as the result of a delocalized sea of electrons being shared among a lattice of positive ions. This description can be a bit misleading, since metals are made of atoms, not ions. However, the aforementioned scenario occurs because the atoms are so close together that their outer electron orbitals overlap, allowing the electrons to move freely among them. Since the negatively charged electrons are no longer attached to a particular atom, the atoms are generally pictured as positive ions with electrons scattered between them, acting as a sort of glue. These bonds give the metallic substance its defined structure, but their strength varies from metal to metal.

Polarity

Polarity is the difference in charge across a compound caused by the uneven partial charge distribution between the atoms. Ionic bonds have higher polarity than covalent bonds because they consist of ions of full opposite charges, meaning one side of the compound is very positive and one very negative. The charge distribution in covalent bonds is more variable, resulting in either polar covalent bonds or non-polar covalent bonds.

NON-POLAR COVALENT BONDS have no uneven distribution of charge. This is because electrons are completely shared between the two atoms, meaning neither has a strong hold on the shared electrons. Non-polar covalent bonds generally arise between two non-metal atoms with equal electronegativity, for example, two hydrogen atoms.

POLAR COVALENT BONDS arise between two non-metal atoms with different electronegativities. In these bonds, electrons are shared unequally. Neither atom is a completely charged ion; instead, the more electronegative atom will hold onto the electron more often, creating a slightly negative charge. The other atom will thus have a slightly negative charge. These slight charges are called DIPOLES.

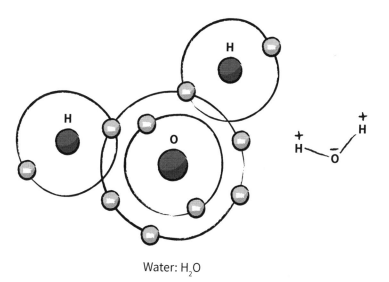

Water: H_2O

Figure 8.5. Polar Covalent Bond

A DIPOLE MOMENT is a measure of the unequal charge distribution in a polar bond. It is possible for a polar molecule to have no net dipole moment if the dipole moments of each bond are equal in magnitude and opposing in direction. These covalent compounds have a symmetrical molecular geometry, meaning that the dipoles created by the polar bond cancel each other out.

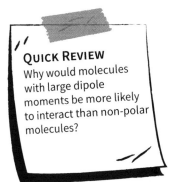

QUICK REVIEW
Why would molecules with large dipole moments be more likely to interact than non-polar molecules?

EXAMPLES

1. Which of the following compounds has highest bond polarity?

    A) NO

    B) CO

    C) H_2

    D) O_2

    B) is correct. Bond polarity increases as the difference in electronegativity between the compounds involved in the bond increases. For molecules composed of two or more atoms of the same type, bonds are non-polar. The distance on the periodic table between carbon and oxygen is greater than the distance between nitrogen and oxygen. Therefore, the electronegativity difference is greater for carbon monoxide, and the bond polarity is therefore also greater.

Intermolecular Bonds

While intramolecular bonds occur within compounds to hold atoms together, it is also possible for bonds to exist between compounds. These intermolecular bonds do not result from the transfer or sharing of electrons. Rather, they are caused by the attraction between the positive and negative parts of separate compounds.

The force of attraction between hydrogen and an extremely electronegative atom, such as oxygen or nitrogen, is known as a HYDROGEN BOND. For example, in water (H_2O), oxygen atoms are attracted to the hydrogen atoms in nearby molecules, creating hydrogen bonds. These bonds are significantly weaker than the chemical bonds that involve sharing or transfer of electrons, and have only 5 to 10 percent of the strength of a covalent bond. Despite its relative weakness, hydrogen bonding is quite important in the natural world; it has major effects on the properties of water and ice and is important biologically with regard to proteins and nucleic acids as well as the DNA double helix structure.

VAN DER WAALS FORCES are electrical interactions between two or more molecules or atoms. They are the weakest type of intermolecular attraction, but if substantial amounts of these forces are present, their net effect can be quite strong.

There are two major types of van der Waals forces. The LONDON DISPERSION FORCE is a temporary force that occurs when electrons in two adjacent atoms form spontaneous, temporary dipoles due to the positions the atoms are occupying. This is the weakest inter-molecular force and it does not exert a force over long distances. Interestingly, London dispersion forces are the only forces that exist between noble gas atoms; without these forces, noble gases would not be able to liquefy.

The second type of van der Waals force is DIPOLE-DIPOLE INTERACTIONS, which are the result of two dipolar molecules interacting with each other. This interaction is simply the partial positive dipole in one molecule being attracted to the partial negative dipole in the other molecule.

EXAMPLES

1. In which of the following molecules are the intermolecular forces strongest?

    A) F_2

    B) I_2

    C) H_2

    D) O_2

    B) is correct. All choices are non-polar molecules with no hydrogen bonding. London dispersion forces are thus the only intermolecular forces present in both of these compounds. The largest molecule will therefore have the strongest intermolecular forces.

2. Which of the following has the highest boiling point?

    A) HF

    B) HI

    C) NaCl

    D) O_2

    A) is correct. Fluorine is a small electronegative atom with which H may form hydrogen bonds. Hydrogen bonds will not arise in any of the remaining molecules, however. Therefore, HF will experience intermolecular forces in the form of hydrogen bonds while the only intermolecular forces present in HI will be dipole-dipole interactions. Since hydrogen bonds are stronger than any other type of intermolecular force, the HF molecules are held close together more tightly than HI molecules, and the substance must be heated to a higher temperature in order to pull the molecules far enough apart from each other to vaporize the substance.

Properties of Substances

Chemical and Physical Properties

Properties of substances are divided into two categories: physical and chemical. PHYSICAL PROPERTIES are those which are measurable and can be seen without changing the chemical makeup of a substance. In contrast, CHEMICAL PROPERTIES are those that determine how a substance will behave in a chemical reaction. These two categories differ in that a physical property may be identified just by observing, touching, or measuring the substance in some way; however, chemical properties cannot by identified simply by observing a material. Rather, the material must be engaged in a chemical reaction in order to identify its chemical properties.

Table 8.3. Physical and Chemical Properties

PHYSICAL PROPERTIES	CHEMICAL PROPERTIES
temperature	heat of combustion
color	flammability
mass	toxicity
viscosity	chemical stability
density	enthalpy of formation

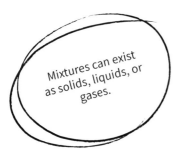

In both physical and chemical changes, matter is always conserved, meaning it can never be created or destroyed.

Mixtures can exist as solids, liquids, or gases.

Mixtures

When substances are combined without a chemical reaction to bond them, the resulting substance is called a MIXTURE. Physical changes can be used to separate mixtures. For example, heating salt water until the water evaporates, leaving the salt behind, will separate a salt water solution.

In a mixture, the components can be unevenly distributed, such as in trail mix or soil. These mixtures are described at HETEROGENEOUS. Alternatively, the components can be HOMOGENOUSLY, or uniformly, distributed, as in salt water. When the distribution is uniform, the mixture is called a SOLUTION. The substance being dissolved is the SOLUTE, and the substance acting on the solute, or doing the dissolving, is the SOLVENT.

Chemical Properties of Water

Though it is one of the most common and biologically essential compounds on Earth, water is chemically abnormal. Its chemical formula is H_2O, which means that water consists of one oxygen atom bound to two hydrogen atoms. The shape of this molecule is often described as looking like Mickey Mouse, with the oxygen atom in the middle as Mickey's face and the two hydrogen atoms as his ears.

This imbalanced shape means that oxygen has a slightly positive charge localized on the two hydrogen atoms, and a slightly negative charge on the lone oxygen. Because of this polarity, water molecules attract each other and tend to clump together, a property called cohension. Water is also extremely adhesive, meaning it clings to other substances. These attractive forces account for a number of water's unique properties.

Water has a high SURFACE TENSION, meaning the bonds between water molecules on the surface of a liquid are stronger than those beneath the surface. Surface tension makes it more difficult to puncture the surface of water. Combined with adhesion, it also helps cause CAPILLARY ACTION, which is the ability of water to travel against gravity. Capillary action moves blood through vessels in the body and water from the roots to the leaves of plants.

As noted earlier, ion substances will dissolve in water. Water is an efficient solvent for ionic compounds because of its hydrogen bonds and associated polarity. When ionic compounds like NaCl are placed in water, the individual ions are attracted to the opposite ends of the dipole moment in water. But water is stronger than the average solvent. In fact, it is known as the "universal solvent," because it is able to dissolve more substances than any other known liquid. The readiness with which ionic compounds dissolve in water is why so many minerals and nutrients are found naturally in water.

Water also has a low molecular weight. Most low-weight compounds exist in a gaseous form at room temperature, but water is a liquid at room temperature. Though water molecules have a relatively low weight, the boiling point and freezing point of water is abnormally high. This is because water's strong hydrogen bonds require high amounts of heat to break. These properties of water make it the only element that is found naturally in all three phases—solid, liquid, and gas—on Earth.

Consistent with its high boiling point, water also has an unusually high specific heat index, meaning that water needs to absorb a lot of heat before it actually gets hot. This property allows the oceans to regulate global temperature, as they can absorb a large amount of energy.

Ice, or frozen water, is also abnormal. Water's hydrogen bonds form a crystalline lattice structure, which puts molecules further apart than usual. Normally, as discussed above, molecules are tightly packed in the solid state. This extra space makes ice less dense than liquid water, which is why ice floats. A solid state being less dense than a liquid state is quite abnormal, but it is also very important for the existence of life on Earth. Because ice is less dense, bodies of water freeze during winter from the top down. Normally they only freeze on the surface, leaving water below for life to continue to flourish.

Osmosis, Diffusion, and Tonicity

Molecules and atoms have a tendency to spread out in space, moving from areas of high concentration to areas of lower concentration. This net movement is called DIFFUSION. When solutions of differing concentrations are separated from each other by a porous

QUICK REVIEW
Consider the unique properties of water, including the fact that solid water is less dense than liquid, the ability of water to act as an efficient solvent, and the high surface tension of water. In what ways do these properties support earth's ecosystems?

membrane, the solute molecules will flow across the membrane in order to equalize these different concentrations. This net movement of solute particles is called OSMOSIS. Osmosis is especially important in biological contexts, as cell and organelle membranes are semi-permeable. Osmosis provides the main means by which water is transported in and out of cells.

When two solutions are separated by a semipermeable membrane, their relative concentrations (which determine the direction of the movement of solute molecules) are called TONICITY. This chemical property is typically used to describe the response of a cell when placed in a solvent.

Three types of tonicity are relevant in biological situations. HYPERTONIC solutions are those which have a higher concentration of a given solute than the interior of the cell. When placed in such solutions, the cell will lose solvent (water) as the solvent travels to areas of higher solute in order to equalize the concentrations. HYPOTONICITY refers to a solution that has a lower concentration of a given solute than the cell. Water will enter the cell, causing it to swell in response to hypotonic solutions. ISOTONIC solutions are those in which solute concentration equals solute concentration inside the cell, and no net flux of solvent will occur between the cell and an isotonic solution.

Hypertonic

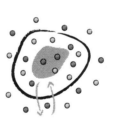
Isotonic

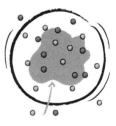
Hypotonic

Figure 8.6. Tonicity

EXAMPLES

1. During times in history when boat travel was common, it was understood among seafarers that saltwater from the ocean was not fit for drinking. Beyond any risk factors associated with purity and cleanliness, what property of saltwater makes it unfit to drink in excessive amounts?

    A) low melting point

    B) high surface tension

    C) hypertonicity

    D) ability of ice to float in water

    C) is correct. Seawater has high concentrations of salts dissolved in it. Consequently, seawater is a hypertonic

States of Matter

All matter exists in one of four **STATES**: solid, liquid, gas, or plasma. **SOLID** matter has densely packed molecules and does not change volume or shape. **LIQUIDS** have more loosely packed molecules and can change shape but not volume. **GAS** molecules are widely dispersed, and gases can change both shape and volume. **PLASMA** is similar to a gas but contains free-moving charged particles (although its overall charge is neutral).

Particles in gases, liquids, and solids all vibrate. Those in gases vibrate and move at high speeds; those in liquids vibrate and move slightly; those in solids vibrate yet stay packed in place in their rigid structure.

Changes in temperature and pressure can cause matter to change states. Generally, adding energy (in the form of heat) changes a substance to a higher energy state (e.g., solid to liquid). Transitions from a high to lower energy state (e.g., liquid to solid) release energy.

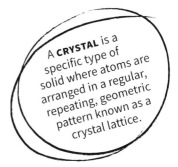

A **CRYSTAL** is a specific type of solid where atoms are arranged in a regular, repeating, geometric pattern known as a crystal lattice.

Each of these changes has a specific name:

- ◆ solid to liquid: melting
- ◆ liquid to solid: freezing
- ◆ liquid to gas: evaporation
- ◆ gas to liquid: condensation
- ◆ solid to gas: sublimation
- ◆ gas to solid: deposition

The occurrence of these processes depends on the amount of energy in individual molecules, rather than the collective energy of the system. For example, in a pool of water outside on a hot day, the whole pool does not evaporate at once; evaporation occurs incrementally in molecules with a high enough energy. Evaporation is also more likely to occur in conjunction with a decrease in the gas pressure around a liquid, since molecules tend to move from areas of high pressure to areas of low pressure.

PHASE DIAGRAMS are used to indicate the phase in which a substance is found at a given pressure and temperature. Phase diagrams are constructed on an *x*, *y*-coordinate system where temperature is plotted along the *x*-axis and pressure is plotted along the y-axis. Phase regions are areas on a phase diagram (corresponding to specific temperature and pressure combinations) at which the substance will exist in a particular physical phase. Lines called phase boundaries separate these phase regions, representing pressure and temperature combinations at which the substance undergoes phase transitions. These are also called lines of equilibrium, because any point on this line represents a pressure and temperature at which multiple phases exist in equilibrium.

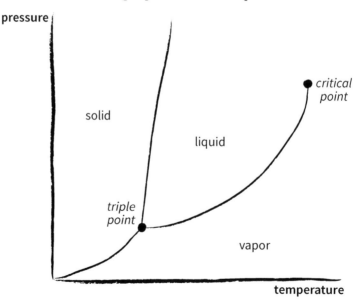

Figure 8.7. Phase Diagram

Every phase diagram includes two important points. The TRIPLE POINT is the point at which the lines of equilibrium intersect and all three phases (solid, liquid, and gas) exist in equilibrium. The second special point on a phase diagram is the CRITICAL POINT. This point is found along the phase boundary between liquid and gas, and is the point at which the phase boundary terminates. This represents the fact that at very high temperature and pressure, liquid and gas phases become indistinguishable. This is known as a supercritical fluid.

Chemical Reactions

A CHEMICAL REACTION involves some sort of chemical change in molecules, atoms, or ions when two or more of these interact. It is important to note that chemical reactions are not the same as state changes. For example, liquid water changing to ice is not a chemical reaction because water and ice have the same chemical properties, just different physical ones. A chemical reaction occurs between two reactants (substances) that form a new substance with different chemical properties than either of the two initial reactants.

REACTANTS are the substances that are consumed or altered in the chemical reaction, while PRODUCTS are substances formed as a result of the chemical reaction. Equations are usually written with the reactants on the left, the products on the right, and an arrow between them. Oftentimes, the arrow has a head on each side, signifying that the reaction occurs in both directions.

Chemical reactions generally occur in two directions. A reaction can move "forward" (for example, two ions combining), and "backward" (for example, an ionic compound separating into its constituent ions). To describe this, chemists say that the reaction occurs in two directions. Most often, catalysts actually serve to accelerate both the forward and reverse reactions. The equilibrium point of a reaction is defined as the point where both the forward and reverse reactions are occurring at equal rates simultaneously—products are turning into reactants and reactants back into products. This produces a state in which, while the reaction is still taking place, no net change in concentration of reactants or products is occurring.

Balancing Chemical Reactions

In the equation below, H_2 and O_2 are the reactants, while water (H_2O) is the product.

$$2H_2 + O_2 \rightarrow 2H_2O$$

In this equation, the number 2 is called a coefficient, and it describes the number of atoms or molecules involved in the reaction. In this reaction, four hydrogen atoms (two molecules of H_2) react with two oxygen atoms. Note that the products also contain four hydrogen and two oxygen molecules. When chemical equations are written, they must include the same number of each atom on both the reactant and product side of the arrow. This is an important step because chemical reactions adhere to the LAW OF CONSERVATION OF MATTER, which states that matter is neither created nor destroyed in a chemical reaction.

In order to balance the equation above, first examine the initial equation without coefficients, which looks like this:

$$H_2 + O_2 \rightarrow H_2O$$

This equation is unbalanced: there are two H atoms on each side, but the reactant side has two O atoms while the product side only has one. To fix this discrepancy, a coefficient of 2 is added in front of the product, H_2O, making the number of O atoms equal on both sides of the equation:

$$H_2 + O_2 \rightarrow 2H_2O$$

Now there are four H atoms on the product side while there are only 2 on the reactant side. This means that in order to finish balancing the equation, a coefficient of 2 must be added in front of H_2, so that there are four H atoms on the reactant side as well:

$$2H_2 + O_2 \rightarrow 2H_2O$$

Remember that in a chemical reaction, only the coefficients may be changed in order to balance it; the subscripts must not be changed. This would be like changing the actual chemical in the equation.

When balancing chemical equations containing atoms of elements in addition to hydrogen and oxygen, wait until the end to balance hydrogen and oxygen atoms.

Types of Reactions

There are several common types of chemical reactions, including decomposition, substitution, and combustion reactions.

DECOMPOSITION reactions are a common class of reaction, consisting of the separation of a compound into atoms or simpler molecules:

General Reaction: $AB \rightarrow A + B$

$$2H_2O_2 \rightarrow 2H_2O + O_2$$

SINGLE SUBSTITUTION reactions are those in which a part of one molecule is replaced by another atom or molecule. Reactivity in single substitutions is determined by the ACTIVITY SERIES, which is a simple list of elements: elements on the list will replace any element that is below it on the list.

General Reaction: $AB + C \rightarrow AC + B$

$$CH_4 + Cl_2 \rightarrow CH_3Cl + HCl$$

Table 8.4. Activity Series

Li	Ca	Mn	Ni	Cu
K	Na	Zn	Sn	Hg
Ba	Mg	Cr	Pb	Ag
Sr	Al	Fe	H_2	Pd
Pt	Au			

In a **DOUBLE SUBSTITUTION** reaction, two parts of two different molecules swap places:

General Reaction: $AB + CD \rightarrow CB + AD$

$$CuCl_2 + 2AgNO_3 \rightarrow Cu(NO_3)_2 + 2AgCl$$

COMBUSTION or burning reactions are high-temperature reactions in which a great deal of heat is released. In combustion reactions, oxygen is a reactant and carbon dioxide and water are produced. Because of the substantial amount of heat energy produced by combustion reactions, they have been important means of generating energy throughout human history, including combustion of fossil fuels, coal, and oil.

General Reaction: $C_xH_x + O_2 \rightarrow CO_2 + H_2O$

$$2C_8H_{18} + 25O_2 \rightarrow 16CO_2 + 18H_2O$$

Reaction Rates

EXOTHERMIC REACTIONS are defined as those which produce energy, whereas **ENDOTHERMIC REACTIONS** need energy in order to occur. Regardless of whether energy is absorbed or released overall, every chemical reaction requires a certain amount of energy in order to begin. This amount is referred to as the **ACTIVATION ENERGY**.

Collisions of reactant particles supply the activation energy for a reaction. The more particles collide, the more energy will be produced. Thus, the more often particles collide, the more likely a reaction is to occur. However, it is quite possible that though some particles collide, not enough energy is generated for an actual reaction to occur.

Given the variability in activation energies of a reaction, as well as variation in the frequency of reactant particle collisions, not all chemical reactions occur at the same rate. A number of variables affect the rate of reaction, including temperature, pressure, concentration, and surface area. The higher the temperature, pressure and concentration, the more likely particles are to collide and thus the reaction rate will be higher. The same is true of surface area for a reaction between a solid and a liquid in which it is immersed. The larger the surface area, the more solid reactant particles are in contact with liquid particles, and the faster the reaction occurs.

EXAMPLES

1. When the following chemical equation for the combustion of methanol (CH_3OH) is balanced, what is the coefficient of H_2O?

   $\_\_CH_3OH + \_\_O_2 \rightarrow \_\_CO_2 + \_\_H_2O$

   A) 3

   B) 2

   C) 1

   D) 4

   B) is correct. To begin balancing a chemical equation, the atoms included in molecules on both sides of the equation must be balanced first. Once these atoms are balanced, move on to balance atoms that appear as reactants or products in their elemental form. In the case of this reaction, C and H are balanced first; O is balanced last. Initially, C is already balanced as one carbon atom is on both the reactant and product sides of the equation. To balance H, add coefficients so that 4 H atoms are on each side of the equation:

   $CH_3OH + O_2 \rightarrow CO_2 + 2H_2O$

   Now, the C, H and O atoms are all balanced, meaning that the same number of each type of atom appears on each side of the equation.

2. How is the following reaction classified?

   $2KClO_3 \rightarrow 2KCl + 3O_2$

   A) decomposition

   B) combustion

   C) substitution

   D) double displacement

   A) is correct. This reaction has a single reactant compound and produces simpler molecules. It is therefore a decomposition reaction.

3. What is the missing product in the following combustion reaction?

$$C_{10}H_8 + 12O_2 \rightarrow H_2O + \underline{}$$

A) CO

B) CH_4

C) CO_2

D) $C_2H_3O_2$

C) is correct. All combustion reactions produce H_2O and CO_2, so the missing product is CO_2.

Catalysts

Catalysts are another factor that can affect reaction rate. **CATALYSTS** reduce the amount of energy that a chemical reaction needs in order to happen, so that the reaction can occur more easily. However, the catalyst itself remains chemically unchanged and is not consumed at all in the reaction. A catalyst lowers the **ACTIVATION ENERGY** for a reaction. It will change the rate of both directions of the reaction, and may change the reaction's equilibrium point as well.

Catalysts function by one of two main methods. The first is **ADSORPTION**, where particles stick to the surface of the catalyst and move around, increasing their likelihood of collision. A more complicated method is the creation of **INTERMEDIATE COMPOUNDS** which are unstable and then break down into other substances, leaving the catalyst in its original state. Many enzymes (proteins which function as catalysts), which are discussed below, work via the creation of intermediate compounds.

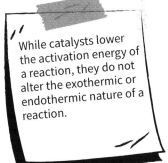

While catalysts lower the activation energy of a reaction, they do not alter the exothermic or endothermic nature of a reaction.

If the rate of a chemical reaction can be increased, it can also be decreased. **INHIBITORS** are essentially the opposite of catalysts, and they act to slow down the reaction rate or even stop the reaction altogether. Inhibitors are used for various reasons, including giving scientists more control over reactions. Both inhibitors and catalysts naturally play significant roles in the chemical reactions that occur in human bodies.

Enzymes

ENZYMES are efficient catalysts functioning in biochemical reactions. They are large, soluble protein molecules that serve to speed up chemical reactions in cells. Cellular respiration, DNA replication, digestion, protein synthesis, and photosynthesis are common processes, all essential for life, that are catalyzed with enzymes.

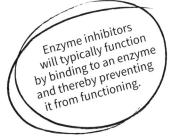

Enzyme inhibitors will typically function by binding to an enzyme and thereby preventing it from functioning.

Like other types of catalysts, enzymes take part in a reaction to provide an alternative pathway with a smaller activation energy, but they remain unchanged themselves. However, enzymes only alter the reaction rate; they do not actually change the equilibrium point of a reaction. Also, unlike most chemical catalysts, enzymes are very selective, which means that they only catalyze certain reactions. (Many other types of catalysts catalyze a variety of reactions.)

This particular aspect of enzyme behavior is referred to as the LOCK AND KEY MODEL. This alludes to the fact that not all keys can open all locks; most keys can only open specific locks. Similarly, the shape of any one enzyme only matches the shape of the molecule it reacts with, called a SUBSTRATE. The ACTIVE SITE is the place on the enzyme that directly contacts the substrate, or the place where the two "puzzle pieces" fit together facilitating the actual reaction.

As suggested by the lock and key model, enzymes are typically highly specific to the reaction they catalyze. In a cellular context, why would it be detrimental if enzymes universally catalyzed any reaction?

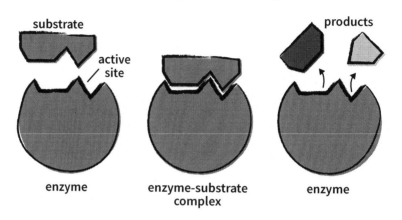

Figure 8.8. Lock and Key Model of Enzymes

Enzymes have a characteristic optimum temperature at which they function best and require a sufficient substrate concentration. At low temperatures, reactions involving enzymes are slow. Conversely, if the temperature is too high, the reaction will slow down and possibly even stop. Generally, enzymes also work most efficiently in neutral conditions rather than in acidic or basic solutions. (One important exception to this is some enzymes that work in the stomach to aid digestion and are optimized to work in very acidic conditions.)

The reason for these restrictions is that variables like temperature and pH affect the shape of an enzyme's active site. In fact, if the temperature is increased too much, usually past 60 degrees Celsius, an enzyme can become DENATURED. This means that the active site has undergone a permanent change in shape, so it can no longer serve its purpose as a catalyst.

EXAMPLES

1. Which of the following statements is true?

   A) Catalysts can "run out."

   B) Catalysts do not participate in chemical reactions.

   C) Enzymes are reactants in biochemical reactions.

   D) An enzyme is effective because it can never be denatured.

   B) is correct. Catalysts are not used up in a chemical reaction, so they cannot run out. Catalysts facilitate chemical reactions, but they do not participate in chemical reactions. Enzymes catalyze biochemical reactions, and as such they do not participate in reactions. Enzymes may be denatured certain conditions just as all proteins may be denatured.

2. Under what conditions do enzyme-catalyzed reactions slow down?

   A) low temperature

   B) low pH

   C) high enzyme concentration

   D) moderately high temperature

   A) is correct. As temperature decreases, the velocity and force with which molecules collide decreases. Thus, there are fewer opportunities for chemical reactions to occur, and the overall rate of reaction decreases.

Acids and Bases

Many scientists have attempted to define and differentiate the properties of acids and bases throughout the centuries. As far back as the sixteenth century, Robert Boyle noted that acids are corrosive, sour, and change the color of vegetable dyes like litmus from blue to red. On the other hand, bases, or alkaline solutions are slippery, bitter, and change the color of litmus from red to blue. The litmus test is still used today to determine whether a solution is acidic or basic.

Later, Svante Arrhenius gave an even more specific definition of acids and bases. He defined ACIDS as compounds that ionize when they dissolve in water, releasing H^+ ions along with a negative ion called a COUNTERION. For example, the well-known acid HCl (hydrochloric acid) dissolves into H^+ and Cl^- ions in water.

Similarly, Arrhenius defined bases as substances which release OH^- ions (hydroxide) and a positive ion when dissolved in water. For example, the compound NaOH dissolves into Na^+ (the counterion) and OH^- ions in water. His theory also explains why acids and bases neutralize each other. If acids have an H^+ ion and bases have an OH^- ion, when combined the ions will form water. Along with the water, the counterions usually combine to form a salt. For example, when HCl and NaOH are combined, the result is water and table salt (H_2O and NaCl).

Despite its simplicity and relevance, there are some faults with Arrhenius' theory of acids and bases. First, since it defines acids and bases by their behavior in water, it only applies to reactions that take place in water. There are also compounds that display basic properties but do not contain the OH^- ion, which presents a problem for defining bases solely based on the fact that they have that ion.

Thomas Lowry and J.N. Bronsted presented a revised theory of acids and bases. In what has been called the Bronsted-Lowry definition of acids and bases, acids are defined as proton donors and bases as proton acceptors. An acid and base are always paired as reactants. The base reactant produces a **CONJUGATE ACID** as a product, paired with a **CONJUGATE BASE** produced from the reactant acid. Water, often involved in these reactions, can either accept or donate a proton, meaning that it can act as either an acid or a base, depending on the particular equation.

In the example below, acetic acid (CH_3CO_2H) is dissolved in water, producing a conjugate base ($CH_3CO_2^-$). Water acts as the base, and its conjugate acid is the hydronium ion (H_3O^+).

$$CH_3CO_2H \quad + \quad H_2O \quad \rightarrow \quad CH_3CO_2^- \quad + \quad H_3O^+$$

$$\text{acid} \qquad\qquad \text{base} \qquad \underset{\text{base}}{\text{conjugate}} \qquad \underset{\text{acid}}{\text{conjugate}}$$

This is perhaps easiest to understand when considering the definition of hydrogen cations. H^+ is essentially a lone proton, and may act as an acid, being donated to another molecule. If it is in a solution of water, it can combine with water to form hydronium, H_3O^+, which is always an acid as it is a proton acceptor.

STRONG ACIDS AND BASES are defined as those that completely ionize in water. Other acids and bases are considered weak, which means that they only partially ionize in water. The strength of an acid or base is measured on the pH scale, which ranges from $1-14$, with 1 being the strongest acid, 14 the strongest base, and 7 being neutral. A substance's pH value is a measure of how many hydrogen ions are in the solution. The scale is exponential, meaning an acid with a pH of 3 has ten times as many hydrogen ions as an acid with a pH of 4. Water, which separates into equal numbers of hydrogen and hydroxide ions, has a neutral pH of 7.

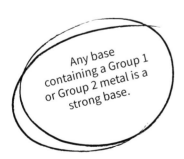

Any base containing a Group 1 or Group 2 metal is a strong base.

Table 8.5. Strong Acids and Bases

STRONG ACIDS	STRONG BASES
HI	NaOH
HBr	KOH
$HClO_4$	LiOH
$HClO_3$	RbOH
HCl	CsOH
HNO_3	$Ca(OH)_2$
$H2SO_4$	$Ba(OH)_2$
	$Sr(OH)_2$

EXAMPLES

1. How is HBr classified in the following reaction?

    $HBr(aq) + KOH(aq) \rightarrow H_3O^+(l) + BrOH(aq)$

    A) acid

    B) base

    C) conjugate acid

    D) conjugate base

    A) is correct. As the reaction occurs in aqueous solution, it is assumed that the reactant and product ionic compounds break into their constituent ions upon dissolving. Thus, the reaction may be written as:

    $H^+ + Br^- + K^+ + OH^- \rightarrow H_3O^+ + Br^- + OH^-$

    When each compound is broken into its constituent ions, it is apparent that HBr donates a proton (H^+) to the OH^- ion to form H_3O^+. Thus, HBr is the acid, KOH is the base and H_3O^+ is the conjugate acid while BrOH is the conjugate base.

2. The following reaction is conventionally written with a single-direction arrow:

    $HCl + NaOH \rightarrow H_2O + NaCl$

    The following reaction, on the other hand, is conventionally written with a double arrow:

    $C_2H_3O_2 + HSO_4^- \leftrightarrow C_2H_2O_2^- + H_2SO_4$

    Why is the first reaction written with a single arrow while the second reaction is written with a double arrow?

    A) The double arrow represents equal product and reactant concentrations.

    B) The double arrow indicates that all reaction components are in the same phase.

    C) The double arrow shows that the reaction is an equilibrium.

    D) The double arrow represents that the reaction is catalyzed.

C) is correct. The first reaction is between a strong acid (HCl) and a strong base (NaOH), which are defined as those which completely ionize in water. Thus, the reverse reaction does not occur, because the reactants will not re-form in aqueous solution. The second reaction is between a weak acid (acetic acid, CH_3COOH) and a weak base (hydrogen sulfate, HSO_4^-). It is clear that these compounds are weak bases because they are not listed in the above table of strong acids and bases. Since weak acids and bases are defined as incompletely ionizing in aqueous solution, the reverse reaction may occur, and so the reaction is written with a double arrow.

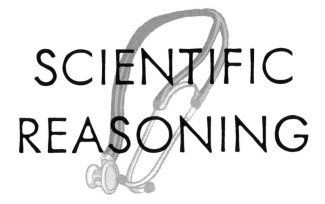

nine

SCIENTIFIC REASONING

The Scientific Method

As developed over thousands of years of painstaking inquiry, the scientific method is a mechanism by which unbiased observations are analyzed and constructed into a testable framework, which is then either preliminarily confirmed or left unsupported.

Properly interpreting results obtained using the scientific method requires acknowledging that scientific endeavors approach the truth—they do not necessarily reveal an irrefutable truth. Thus, previous scientific findings that have been subsequently corrected should not be considered erroneous; rather they should be viewed as less accurate than determinations made using improved technology and methodology. Similarly, current medical views are not only subject to change but almost certain to change as medical science advances.

Utility of the scientific method is by no means restricted to professional scientists. Its principles are of particular importance to medical practitioners, who must impartially observe symptoms, form a preliminary diagnosis, and verify its accuracy. Medical practitioners must employ scientific medical knowledge to properly treat maladies and assess the effectiveness of these treatments. As such, a proper understanding of the scientific method is paramount for medical practitioners at all stages.

In brief, the scientific method involves several sequential stages, and the reliability of each stage is contingent on the reliability of the preceding stages. First, **OBSERVATIONS** are made in as unbiased a manner as possible. In evaluating medical treatments, this often involves "blinding" both practitioners and patients to the experimental group identity of participants (a "double-blind" experimental design). Blinding ensures that the expectations of the patients do not affect the outcomes of their treatment (potentially resulting in a placebo effect) and that the expectations of the practitioners do not bias the interpretation of the results.

The observations are then evaluated in the context of existing medical knowledge of the disease and its treatment. This will properly determine the treatment efficacy and possibly its mechanism of action in cases when the effects of the treatment are not thoroughly understood. These observations are then formed into a HYPOTHESIS, a specific testable question regarding the treatment or disease etiology. Critically, this hypothesis must be falsifiable; in other words, if a hypothesis cannot feasibly be disproven by scientifically rigorous testing, it is invalid scientifically.

The hypothesis is then TESTED through a carefully designed experiment or trial. It is important to eliminate confounding variables in experimental design. For example, a cardiac drug may be given to patients in a trial, while a placebo is given to healthy control individuals. If the controls are considerably older than the patients, this may artificially bias some outcome measures of the trial to make the drug seem more effective than it would otherwise appear.

Finally, the aggregate results of experiments may be constructed into a working THEORY relating to the etiology of a disease or its treatment. The term *theory* implies that while understanding of a concept is still developing and subject to change, it is heavily supported by multiple lines of evidence. For example, the notion that following proper sterile procedures is essential to avoid infection following medical procedures arises from the germ theory of disease. An overwhelming amount of data support this understanding of disease pathology, so using the word *theory* implies that it is very likely that germs cause infection, while still leaving some room for doubt.

Designing Experiments

Designing a medical study may entail using the scientific method itself to develop foundational knowledge for further advancement in the experimental process. For example, investigators might develop a HYPOTHESIS-SEEKING study for a poorly understood disease or treatment. They might predict that a treatment would induce changes to gene expression, without knowing which genes will be affected. Once some information is gleaned about a particular disease or treatment, a HYPOTHESIS-DRIVEN investigation might be undertaken, in which investigators test a particular hypothesis (e.g. "because we know that this treatment affects gene X, and gene

X is related to the cause of this disease, we predict that regulating gene X might be essential for the treatment to be effective").

Scientists use a rigorous set of rules to design experiments. The protocols of experimental design are meant to ensure that scientists are actually testing what they set out to test. A well-designed experiment will measure the impact of a single factor on a system, thus allowing the experimenter to draw conclusions about that factor.

Every experiment includes variables, which are the factors that may impact the outcome of the experiment. INDEPENDENT VARIABLES are controlled by the experimenter. They are usually the factors that the experimenter has hypothesized will have an effect on the system. Often, a design will include a treatment group and a CONTROL GROUP (which does not receive the treatment). The DEPENDENT VARIABLES are factors that are influenced by the independent variable.

For example, in an experiment investigating which type of fertilizer has the greatest effect on plant growth, the independent variable is the type of fertilizer used. The scientist is controlling, or manipulating, the type of fertilizer. The dependent variable is plant growth because the amount of plant growth depends on the type of fertilizer. The type of plant, the amount of water, and the amount of sunlight the plants receive are controls because those variables of the experiment are kept the same for each plant.

What are the limitations of adhering rigidly to the scientific method?

When designing an experiment, scientists must identify possible sources of error. These can be CONFOUNDING VARIABLES, which are factors that act like the independent variable and thus can make it appear that the independent variable has a greater effect than it actually does. The design may also include unknown variables that are not controlled by the scientists. Finally, scientists must be aware of human error, particularly in collecting data and making observations, and of possible equipment errors.

During the experiment, scientists collect data, which must then be analyzed and presented appropriately. This may mean running a statistical analysis on the data (e.g., finding the mean) or putting the data in graph form. Such an analysis allows scientists to see trends in the data and determine if those trends are statistically significant. From that data, scientists can draw a CONCLUSION about the experiment.

Scientists often use MODELS in their research. These models are a simplified representation of a system. For example, a mathematical equation that describes fluctuations in a population might be used to test how a certain variable is likely to affect that population. Or, a scientist might use a greenhouse to model a particular ecosystem so that she or he can more closely control the variables in the environment.

The path from the initial investigation of a disease or treatment to the development of new therapeutics is often extremely long, involving many teams of researchers over many years. PRECLINICAL STUDIES attempt to determine the causes of disease and how they might be reduced or reversed. TRANSLATIONAL STUDIES apply the findings of the earlier research to clinically relevant situations, often examining whether findings in animals are also relevant in human clinical populations.

Once a clear effect and mechanism of a potential treatment has been demonstrated, a novel drug might enter CLINICAL TRIALS. These trials occur in four phases (I–IV). PHASE I trials evaluate the safety of the drug and optimize dosage. If the drug is sufficiently safe, it enters PHASE II, wherein it is evaluated for efficacy, often in contrast to existing treatments; safety is also examined. Sufficiently safe and effective drugs enter PHASE III, when a larger group of patients is administered the drug in order to confirm safety and efficacy. Groups that succeed in Phase III may be approved by regulatory bodies, and at that point they can be marketed and prescribed for the general population. Finally, once a drug has been made available, PHASE IV trials evaluate the effects of long-term usage of the drug and determine if its effects vary between different patient populations. Even at the clinical trial stage, it may be years before a potential treatment is applied in general clinical practice, and many potential treatments are not approved for usage due to their performance in these rigorous examinations of safety and efficacy.

EXAMPLES

1. Why is a double-blind study design valuable in clinical studies?

    A) It reduces costs.

    B) It allows for observations to be made.

    C) It creates a placebo effect.

    D) It prevents producing biased data.

    D) is correct. A double-blind study design can prevent the expectations of both the patient and clinician from biasing the data.

2. Why is the germ theory of disease considered to be a theory?

    A) There is insufficient evidence to support it.

    B) Valid alternative explanations exist.

    C) Although not irrefutably proven, it is strongly supported by existing evidence.

    D) It has only limited clinical application.

C) is correct. A scientific theory is typically strongly supported by evidence, despite public misunderstanding to the contrary.

3. A team of investigators wants to address the question, "which genes within the hippocampus are altered in the context of depression?" Their methods are focused around large-scale genetic screening of as many genes as possible throughout the genome. Which of the following best describes this type of investigation?

   A) hypothesis-driven

   B) hypothesis-seeking

   C) hypothesis-related

   D) Phase I clinical trial

   B) is correct. This hypothetical investigation would be hypothesis-seeking, as the team hopes to generate potential target genes to guide subsequent experiments.

4. A team of investigators wants to address the question, "if expression of [a particular gene] is reduced in the brains of depressed patients, will increasing levels of this particular molecule reduce depressive symptoms?" Which of the following best describes this type of investigation?

   A) hypothesis-driven

   B) hypothesis-seeking

   C) hypothesis-related

   D) Phase I clinical trial

   A) is correct. This design aims to investigate a specific hypothesis based on previous evidence.

5. A new drug has been shown to potentially reduce symptoms in a particular disorder, and its safety is assessed to determine if it might be valid to prescribe to patients. Which of the following best describes this type of investigation?

   A) hypothesis-driven

   B) hypothesis-seeking

   C) hypothesis-related

   D) Phase I clinical trial

   D) is correct. This investigation meets the specific criteria of a Phase 1 clinical trial.

PART IV: ENGLISH AND LANGUAGE USE

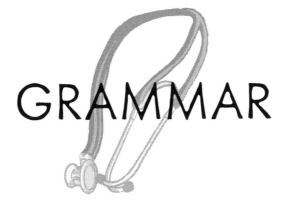

ten

GRAMMAR

G RAMMAR refers to the structures and systems that make up a language. The TEAS will test your ability to identify important grammatical terms and to use conventional rules of grammar to craft sentences that are correct, clear, and concise.

Parts of Speech

The **PARTS OF SPEECH** are the building blocks of sentences, paragraphs, and entire texts. Grammarians have typically defined eight parts of speech—nouns, pronouns, verbs, adverbs, adjectives, conjunctions, prepositions, and interjections—all of which play unique roles in the context of a sentence. Thus, a fundamental understanding of the parts of speech is necessary in order to form an understanding of basic sentence construction.

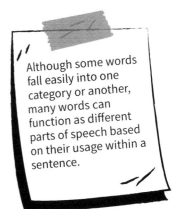

Although some words fall easily into one category or another, many words can function as different parts of speech based on their usage within a sentence.

Nouns and Pronouns

NOUNS are the words we use to give names to people, places, things, and ideas. Most often, nouns fill the position of subject or object within a sentence. The category of NOUNS has several subcategories: common nouns (*chair, car, house*), proper nouns (*Julie, David*), abstract nouns (*love, intelligence, sadness*), concrete nouns (*window, bread, person*), compound nouns (*brother-in-law, rollercoaster*), non-countable nouns (*money, water*), countable nouns (*dollars, cubes*), and verbal nouns (*writing, diving*). There is much crossover between these subcategories (for example, *chair* is common, concrete, and countable).

Sometimes, a word that is typically used as a noun will be used to modify another noun. The word then would be labeled as an adjective because of its usage within the sentence. In the following example, *cabin* is a noun in the first sentence and an adjective in the second:

The family visited the <u>cabin</u> by the lake.

Our <u>cabin</u> stove overheated during vacation.

PRONOUNS replace nouns in a sentence or paragraph, allowing a writer to achieve a smooth flow throughout a text by avoiding unnecessary repetition. The unique aspect of the pronoun as a part of speech is that the list of pronouns is finite: while there are innumerable nouns in the English language, the list of pronouns is rather limited in contrast. The noun that a pronoun replaces is called its **ANTECEDENT**.

Pronouns fall into several distinct categories. **PERSONAL PRONOUNS** act as subjects or objects in a sentence:

<u>She</u> received a letter; I gave the letter to <u>her</u>.

POSSESSIVE PRONOUNS indicate possession:

<u>My</u> coat is red; <u>our</u> car is blue.

REFLEXIVE (intensive) **PRONOUNS** intensify a noun or reflect back upon a noun:

I <u>myself</u> made the dessert. I made the dessert <u>myself</u>.

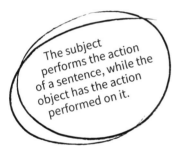

The subject performs the action of a sentence, while the object has the action performed on it.

Personal, possessive, and reflexive pronouns must all agree with the noun that they replace both in gender (male, female, or neutral), number (singular or plural), and person. **PERSON** refers to the point of view of the sentence. First person is the point of view of the speaker (I, me), second person is the person being addressed (you), and third person refers to a person outside the sentence (he, she, they).

Table 10.1. Personal, Possessive, and Reflexive Pronouns

CASE	FIRST PERSON		SECOND PERSON		THIRD PERSON	
	singular	plural	singular	plural	singular	plural
subject	I	we	you	you (all)	he, she, it,	they
object	me	us	you	you (all)	him, her, it	them
possessive	my	our	your	your	his, her, its	their
reflexive	myself	our-selves	yourself	your-selves	himself, herself, itself	them-selves

RELATIVE PRONOUNS begin dependent clauses. Like other pronouns, they may appear in subject or object case, depending on the clause. Take, for example, the sentence below:

Charlie, <u>who</u> made the clocks, works in the basement.

Here, the relative pronoun *who* is substituting for Charlie; that word indicates that Charlie makes the clocks, and so *who* is in the subject case because it is performing the action (*makes the clocks*).

In cases where a person is the object of a relative clause, the writer would use the relative pronoun *whom*. For example, read the sentence below:

My father, <u>whom</u> I care for, is sick.

Even though *my father* is the subject of the sentence, in the relative clause the relative pronoun *whom* is the object of the preposition *for*. Therefore that pronoun appears in the object case.

When a relative clause refers to a non-human, *that* or *which* is used. (*I live in Texas, <u>which</u> is a large state.*) The relative pronoun *whose* indicates possession. (*I don't know <u>whose</u> car that is.*)

Table 10.2. Relative Pronouns

PRONOUN TYPE	SUBJECT	OBJECT
person	who	whom
thing	which, that	
possessive	whose	

INTERROGATIVE PRONOUNS begin questions (*<u>Who</u> worked last evening?*). They request information about people, places, things, ideas, location, time, means, and purposes.

Table 10.3. Interrogative Pronouns

INTERROGATIVE PRONOUN	ASKS ABOUT	EXAMPLE
who	person	<u>Who</u> lives there?
whom	person	To <u>whom</u> shall I send the letter?
what	thing	<u>What</u> is your favorite color?
where	place	<u>Where</u> do you go to school?
when	time	<u>When</u> will we meet for dinner?
which	selection	<u>Which</u> movie would you like to see?
why	reason	<u>Why</u> are you going to be late?
how	manner	<u>How</u> did the ancient Egyptians build the pyramids?

DEMONSTRATIVE PRONOUNS point out or draw attention to something or someone. They can also indicate proximity or distance.

Table 10.4. Demonstrative Pronouns

Number	Subject/ Proximity	Example	Object/ Distance	Example
singular	this (subject)	This is my apart-ment—please come in!	that (object)	I gave that to him yesterday.
	this (proximity)	This is the com-puter you will use right here, not the one in the other office.	that (distance)	That is the Statue of Liberty across the harbor.
plural	these (subject)	These are flaw-less diamonds.	those (object)	Give those to me later.
	these (proximity)	These right here are the books we want, not the ones over there.	those (distance)	Those mountains across the plains are called the Rockies.

Indefinite pronouns simply replace nouns to avoid unnecessary repetition:

Several came to the party to see both.

Indefinite pronouns can be either singular or plural (and some can act as both depending on the context). If the indefinite pronoun is the subject of the sentence, it is important to know whether that pronoun is singular or plural so that the verb can agree with the pronoun in number.

Table 10.5. Common Indefinite Pronouns

singular	another, anybody, anyone, any-thing, each, either, everybody, everyone, everything, neither, no one, nobody, nothing, one, some-body, someone, something
plural	both, few, many, several
singular or plural	all, any, some, more, most, none*

*These pronouns take their singularity or plurality from the object of the preposi-tions that follow: Some of the pies were eaten. Some of the pie was eaten.

Verbs

VERBS express action (*run, jump, play*) or state of being (*is, seems*). The former are called action verbs, and the latter are linking verbs. Linking verbs join the subject of the sentence to the subject com-plement, which follows the verb and provides more information about the subject. See the sentence below:

The dog is cute.

The dog is the subject, *is* is the linking verb, and *cute* is the subject complement.

Verbs can stand alone or they can be accompanied by HELPING VERBS, which are used to indicate tense. Verb tense indicates the time of the action. The action may have occurred in the past, present, or future. The action may also have been simple (occurring once) or continuous (ongoing). The perfect and perfect continuous tenses describe when actions occur in relation to other actions.

Table 10.6. Verb Tenses

TENSE	PAST	PRESENT	FUTURE
simple	I answered the question.	I answer your questions in class.	I will answer your question.
continuous	I was answering your question when you interrupted me.	I am answering your question; please listen.	I will be answering your question after the lecture.
perfect	I had answered all questions before class ended.	I have answered the questions already.	I will have answered every question before the class is over.
perfect continuous	I had been answering questions when the students started leaving.	I have been answering questions for 30 minutes and am getting tired.	I will have been answering students' questions for 20 years by the time I retire.

Helping Verbs: is/am/are/was/were, be/being/been, has/had/have, do/does/did, might, may, can, should, would, could, shall, must, will

Changing the spelling of the verb and/or adding helping verbs is known as CONJUGATION. In addition to being conjugated for tense, verbs are conjugated to indicate *person* (first, second, and third person) and *number* (whether they are singular or plural). The conjugation of the verb must agree with the subject of the sentence. A verb that has not been conjugated is called an infinitive and begins with *to* (*to swim, to be*).

Table 10.7. Verb Conjugation (Present Tense)

PERSON	SINGULAR	PLURAL
first person	I answer	we answer
second person	you answer	you (all) answer
third person	he/she/it answers	they answer

Verbs may be regular, meaning they follow normal conjugation patterns, or irregular, meaning they do not follow a regular pattern.

Table 10.8. Regular and Irregular Verbs

	Simple Present	Present Participle	Simple Past	Past Participle
Regular	help	helping	helped	(have) helped
	jump	jumping	jumped	(have) jumped
Irregular	am	been	was	(have) been
	swim	swimming	swam	(have) swum
	sit	sitting	sat	(have) sat
	set	setting	set	(have) set
	lie	lying	lay	(have) lain
	lay	laying	laid	(have) laid
	rise	rising	rose	(have) risen
	raise	raising	raised	(have) raised

Verbs can be written in the active or passive voice. In the ACTIVE VOICE, the subject of the sentence performs the main action of the sentence. In the sentence below, Alexis is performing the action:

Alexis played tennis.

In the passive voice, the subject of the sentence is receiving the action of the main verb. In the sentence below, the subject is *tennis*, which receives the action *played*:

Tennis was played.

Note that, in the passive voice, there is no indication of who performed the action. For this reason, passive voice is used when the subject is unknown or unimportant. For example, in science, it is common to use the passive voice:

The experiment was performed three times.

At most other times, it is considered more appropriate to use the active voice because it is more dynamic and gives more information.

Finally, verbs can be classified by whether they take a DIRECT OBJECT, which is a noun that receives the action of the verb. Transitive verbs require a direct object. In the sentence below, the transitive verb *throw* has a direct object (ball):

The pitcher will throw <u>the ball</u>.

Intransitive verbs do not require a direct object. Verbs like *run*, *jump*, and *go* make sense without any object:

He will run.

She jumped.

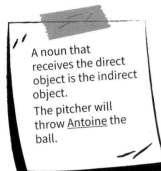

A noun that receives the direct object is the indirect object.

The pitcher will throw <u>Antoine</u> the ball.

Many sets of similar verbs include one transitive and one intransitive verb, which can cause confusion. These troublesome verbs include combinations such as *lie* or *lay*, *rise* or *raise*, and *sit* or *set*.

Table 10.9. Intransitive and Transitive Verbs

INTRANSITIVE VERBS	TRANSITIVE VERBS
lie – to recline	lay – to put (lay <u>something</u>)
rise – to go or get up	raise – to lift (raise <u>something</u>)
sit – to be seated	set – to put (set <u>something</u>)
Hint: These intransitive verbs have *i* as the second letter. *Intransitive* begins with *i*.	Hint: The word *transitive* begins with a *t*, and it *TAKES* an object.

EXAMPLES

Choose the correct verb from the two choices:

1. (Lying/laying) in the basket, the flowers dried beautifully.

    <u>Lying</u> in the basket, the flowers dried beautifully.

2. We (sat/set) the ladder upright.

    We <u>set</u> the ladder upright.

3. (Rise/Raise) early at dawn to see the pigs.

    <u>Rise</u> early at dawn to see the pigs.

Adjectives and Adverbs

ADVERBS take on a modifying or describing role and often take the ending *–ly*. These words can describe a number of different parts of speech and even phrases or clauses:

- verbs: *He <u>quickly</u> ran to the house next door.*
- adjectives: *Her <u>very</u> effective speech earned her a new job.*
- other adverbs: *Several puppies arrived <u>rather</u> happily after they had eaten dog treats.*
- entire sentences: *<u>Instead</u>, the owner kept his shop.*

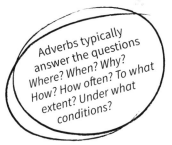

Adverbs typically answer the questions Where? When? Why? How? How often? To what extent? Under what conditions?

Like adverbs, **ADJECTIVES** modify or describe, but they add to the meaning of nouns and pronouns only:

<u>Five thoughtful</u> students came to work at the farm.

The idea from the committee proved a <u>smart</u> one.

One very important note regarding the adjective is that any word used to describe a noun or pronoun will be classified as an adjective. *Her* could be used as a pronoun or an adjective depending on usage:

<u>Her</u> dog barks until midnight. (adjective modifying *dog*)

We gave several books to <u>her</u>. (pronoun)

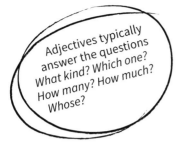

Adjectives typically answer the questions What kind? Which one? How many? How much? Whose?

Also note that *a*, *and*, and *the* (called articles) are always adjectives.

Conjunctions

CONJUNCTIONS join words into phrases, clauses, and sentences by use of three mechanisms. There are three main types of conjunctions. COORDINATING CONJUNCTIONS join together two independent clauses (i.e., two complete thoughts). These include *and*, *but*, *or*, *for*, *nor*, *yet*, *so* (FANBOYS). Note that some of these can also be used to join items in a series.

I'll order lunch, <u>but</u> you need to go pick it up.

Make sure to get sandwiches, chips, <u>and</u> sodas.

CORRELATIVE CONJUNCTIONS (whether/or, either/or, neither/nor, both/and, not only/but also) work together to join items:

<u>Both</u> the teacher <u>and</u> the students needed a break after the lecture.

SUBORDINATING CONJUNCTIONS join dependent clauses (thoughts that cannot stand alone as sentences) to the related independent clause. They usually describe some sort of relationship between the two parts of the sentence, such as cause/effect or order. They can appear at the beginning or in the middle of a sentence:

We treat ourselves during football season to several orders <u>because</u> we love pizza.

<u>Because</u> we love pizza, we treat ourselves during football season to several orders.

Table 10.10. Subordinating Conjunctions

time	after, as, as long as, as soon as, before, since, until, when, whenever, while
manner	as, as if, as though
cause	because
condition	although, as long as, even if, even though, if, provided that, though, unless, while
purpose	in order that, so that, that
comparison	as, than

When using correlative conjunctions, be sure that the structure of the word, phrase, or clause that follows the first part of the conjunction mirrors the structure of the word, phrase, or clause that follows the second part.

Correct: I will neither <u>mow the grass</u> nor <u>pull the weeds</u> today.

Incorrect: I will neither <u>mow the grass</u> nor <u>undertake the pulling of the weeds</u> today.

Prepositions

PREPOSITIONS set up relationships in time (*after the party*) or space (*under the cushions*) within a sentence. A preposition will always function as part of a prepositional phrase, which includes the preposition along with the object of the preposition. If a word that usually acts as a preposition is standing alone in a sentence, the word is likely functioning as an adverb:

She hid <u>underneath</u>.

Table 10.11 Common Prepositions

PREPOSITIONS	COMPOUND PREPOSITIONS
along, among, around, at, before, behind, below, beneath, beside, besides, between, beyond, by, despite, down, during, except, for, from, in, into, near, of, off, on, onto, out, outside, over, past, since, through, till, to, toward, under, underneath, until, up, upon, with, within, without	according to, as of, as well as, aside from, because of, by means of, in addition to, in front of, in place of, in respect to, in spite of, instead of, on account of, out of, prior to, with regard to

Interjections

INTERJECTIONS have no grammatical attachment to the sentence itself other than to add expressions of emotion. These parts of speech may be punctuated with commas or exclamation points and may fall anywhere within the sentence itself:

<u>Ouch</u>! He stepped on my toe.

She shopped at the stores after Christmas and, <u>hooray</u>, found many items on sale.

I have seen his love for his father in many expressions of concern—<u>Wow</u>!

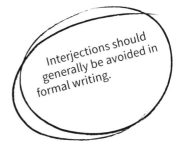

Interjections should generally be avoided in formal writing.

EXAMPLES

1. List all of the adjectives used in the following sentence:

Her camera fell into the turbulent water, so her frantic friend quickly grabbed the damp item.

A) turbulent, frantic, damp

B) turbulent, frantic, quickly, damp

C) her, turbulent, her, frantic, damp

D) her, the, turbulent, her, frantic, the, damp

D) is correct. *Turbulent*, *frantic*, and *damp* are adjectives; *her* is modifying first *camera* and then *friend*; and *the* is always a limiting adjective—the definite article.

2. List all of the pronouns used in the following sentence:

Several of the administrators who had spoken clearly on the budget increase gave both of the opposing committee members a list of their ideas.

A) several, of, their

B) several, who, both

C) several, who, both, their

D) several, both

B) is correct. *Several* is an indefinite plural pronoun; *who* is a relative pronoun introducing the adjectival clause *who had spoken clearly on the budget increase*; *both* is an indefinite plural pronoun.

3. List all of the conjunctions in the following sentence, and indicate after each conjunction whether it's coordinating, correlative, or subordinating:

The political parties do not know if the most popular candidates will survive until the election, but neither the voters nor the candidates will give up their push for popularity.

A) if (subordinating), until (subordinating), but (coordinating), neither/nor (correlative), for (coordinating)

B) if (subordinating), but (coordinating), neither/nor (correlative), for (coordinating)

C) if (subordinating), but (coordinating), neither/nor (correlative)

D) if (subordinating), until (subordinating), but (coordinating), neither/nor (correlative), up (subordinating), for (coordinating)

C) is correct. *If* is acting as a subordinating conjunction; *but* is acting as a coordinating conjunction; and *neither/nor* is a correlative conjunction pair.

Constructing Sentences

SYNTAX is the study of how words are combined to create sentences. In English, words are used to build phrases and clauses, which, in turn, are combined to create sentences. By varying the order and length of phrases and clauses, writers can create sentences that are diverse and interesting.

Phrases and clauses are made up of either a subject, a predicate, or both. The **SUBJECT** is what the sentence is about. It will be a noun that is usually performing the main action of the sentence, and it may be accompanied by modifiers. The **PREDICATE** describes what the subject is doing or being. It contains the verb(s) and any modifiers or objects that accompany it.

Phrases

A **PHRASE** is a group of words that communicates a partial idea and lacks either a subject or a predicate. Several phrases may be strung together, one after another, to add detail and interest to a sentence.

The animals crossed <u>the large bridge to eat the fish on the wharf</u>.

Phrases are categorized based on the main word in the phrase. A **PREPOSITIONAL PHRASE** begins with a preposition and ends with an object of the preposition; a **VERB PHRASE** is composed of the main verb along with its helping verbs; and a **NOUN PHRASE** consists of a noun and its modifiers.

prepositional phrase: The dog is hiding <u>under the porch</u>.

verb phrase: The chef <u>would have created</u> another soufflé, but the staff protested.

noun phrase: <u>The big, red barn</u> rests beside <u>the vacant chicken house</u>.

An **APPOSITIVE PHRASE** is a particular type of noun phrase that renames the word or group of words that precedes it. Appositive phrases usually follow the noun they describe and are set apart by commas.

My dad, <u>a clock maker</u>, loved antiques.

VERBAL PHRASES begin with a word that would normally act as a verb but is instead filling another role within the sentence. These phrases can act as nouns, adjectives, or adverbs. **GERUND PHRASES** begin with gerunds, which are verbs that end in *–ing* and act as nouns.

gerund phrase: <u>Writing numerous Christmas cards</u> occupies her aunt's time each year.

A **PARTICIPIAL PHRASE** is a verbal phrase that acts as an adjective. These phrases start with either present participles (which end in *–ing*) or past participles (which usually end in *–ed*). Participial phrases can be extracted from the sentence, and the sentence will still make sense because the participial phrase is playing only a modifying role:

<u>Enjoying the stars that filled the sky</u>, Dave lingered outside for quite a while.

The word *gerund* has an *n* in it, a helpful reminder that the gerund acts as a noun. Therefore, the gerund phrase might act as the subject, the direct object, or the object of the preposition just as another noun would.

Finally, an INFINITIVE PHRASE is a verbal phrase that may act as a noun, an adjective, or an adverb. Infinitive phrases begin with the word *to*, followed by a simple form of a verb (to eat, to jump, to skip, to laugh, to sing).

<u>To visit Europe</u> had always been her dream.

Clauses

CLAUSES contain both a subject and a predicate. They can be either independent or dependent. An INDEPENDENT (or main) CLAUSE can stand alone as its own sentence:

The dog ate her homework.

Dependent (or subordinate) clauses cannot stand alone as their own sentences. They start with a subordinating conjunction, relative pronoun, or relative adjective, which will make them sound incomplete:

<u>Because</u> the dog ate her homework

Table 10.12. Words That Begin Dependent Clauses

SUBORDINATING CONJUNCTIONS	RELATIVE PRONOUNS AND ADJECTIVES
after, before, once, since, until, when, whenever, while, as, because, in order that, so, so that, that, if, even if, provided that, unless, although, even though, though, whereas, where, wherever, than, whether	who, whoever, whom, whomever, whose, which, that, when, where, why, how

Types of Sentences

Sentences can be classified based on the number and type of clauses they contain. A SIMPLE SENTENCE will have only one independent clause and no dependent clauses. The sentence may contain phrases, complements, and modifiers, but it will comprise only one independent clause, one complete idea.

The cat under the back porch jumped against the glass yesterday.

A COMPOUND SENTENCE has two or more independent clauses and no dependent clauses:

The cat under the back porch jumped against the glass yesterday, and he scared my grandma.

A COMPLEX SENTENCE has only one independent clause and one or more dependent clauses:

The cat under the back porch, who loves tuna, jumped against the glass yesterday.

A COMPOUND-COMPLEX SENTENCE has two or more independent clauses and one or more dependent clause:

The cat under the back porch, who loves tuna, jumped against the glass yesterday; he left a mark on the window.

Table 10.13. Sentence Structure and Clauses

SENTENCE STRUCTURE	INDEPENDENT CLAUSES	DEPENDENT CLAUSES
simple	1	0
compound	2 +	0
complex	1	1 +
compound-complex	2 +	1 +

Writers can diversify their use of phrases and clauses in order to introduce variety into their writing. Variety in SENTENCE STRUCTURE not only makes writing more interesting but also allows writers to emphasize that which deserves emphasis. In a paragraph of complex sentences, a short, simple sentence can be a powerful way to draw attention to a major point.

EXAMPLES

1. Identify the prepositional phrase in the following sentence:

   Wrapping packages for the soldiers, the kind woman tightly rolled the t-shirts to see how much space remained for the homemade cookies.

   A) Wrapping packages for the soldiers

   B) the kind woman

   C) to see how much space

   D) for the homemade cookies

   D) is correct. This phrase begins with the preposition *for*.

2. Which sentence is correct in its sentence structure label?

   A) The grandchildren and their cousins enjoyed their day at the beach. (compound)

   B) Most of the grass has lost its deep color despite the fall lasting into December. (complex)

   C) The members who had served selflessly were cheering as the sequestration ended. (simple)

   D) Do as you please. (complex)

   D) is correct. This sentence is complex because it has one independent clause (*Do*) and one dependent (*as you please*).

Punctuation

Many of the choices writers must make relate to **PUNCTUATION**. While creative writers have the liberty to play with punctuation to achieve their desired ends, academic and technical writers must adhere to stricter conventions. The main punctuation marks are periods, question marks, exclamation marks, colons, semi-colons, commas, quotation marks, and apostrophes.

There are three terminal punctuation marks that can be used to end sentences. The **PERIOD** is the most common and is used to end declarative (statement) and imperative (command) sentences. The **QUESTION MARK** is used to end interrogative sentences, and exclamation marks are used to indicate that the writer or speaker is exhibiting intense emotion or energy.

Sarah and I are attending a concert.

How many people are attending the concert?

What a great show that was!

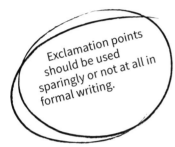

Exclamation points should be used sparingly or not at all in formal writing.

The **COLON** and the **SEMI-COLON**, though often confused, have a unique set of rules surrounding their respective uses. While both punctuation marks are used to join clauses, the construction of the clauses and the relationship between them varies.

The **SEMI-COLON** is used to show a general relationship between two independent clauses (IC; IC):

The disgruntled customer tapped angrily on the counter; she had to wait nearly ten minutes to speak to the manager.

Coordinating conjunctions (FANBOYS) cannot be used with semi-colons. However, conjunctive adverbs can be used following a semi-colon:

She may not have to take the course this <u>year; however,</u> she will eventually have to sign up for that specific course.

The **COLON**, somewhat less limited than the semi-colon in its usage, is used to introduce a list, definition, or clarification. While the clause preceding the colon must be an independent clause, the clause that follows does not have to be one:

Incorrect. The buffet offers three choices that include: ham, turkey, or roast.

Correct. The buffet offers three choices: ham, turkey, or roast.

Correct. The buffet offers three choices that include the following: ham, turkey, or roast.

Note that neither the semi-colon nor the colon should be used to set off an introductory phrase from the rest of the sentence.

Incorrect. After the trip to the raceway; we realized that we should have brought ear plugs.

Incorrect. After the trip to the raceway: we realized that we should have brought ear plugs.

Correct. After the trip to the raceway, we realized that we should have brought ear plugs.

The COMMA is a complicated piece of punctuation that can serve many different purposes within a sentence. Many times comma placement is an issue of style, not mechanics, meaning there is not necessarily one correct way to write the sentence. There are, however, a few important hard-and-fast comma rules to be followed.

Many people are taught that a comma represents a pause for breath. While this trick is useful for helping young readers, it is not a helpful guide for comma usage when writing.

1. Commas should be used to separate two independent clauses along with a coordinating conjunction.

   George ordered the steak, but Bruce preferred the ham.

2. Commas should be used to separate coordinate adjectives (two different adjectives that describe the same noun).

   The shiny, regal horse ran majestically through the wide, open field.

3. Commas should be used to separate items in a series. The comma before the conjunction is called the Oxford or serial comma, and is optional.

   The list of groceries included cream, coffee, donuts, and tea.

4. Commas should be used to separate introductory words, phrases, and clauses from the rest of the sentence.

   Slowly, Nathan became aware of his surroundings after the concussion.

   Within an hour, the authorities will descend on the home.

   After Alice swam the channel, nothing intimidated her.

5. Commas should be used to set off non-essential information and appositives.

   Estelle, our newly elected chairperson, will be in attendance.

   Ida, my neighbor, watched the children for me last week.

6. Commas should be used to set off titles of famous individuals.

Charles, Prince of Wales, visited Canada several times in the last ten years.

7. Commas should be used to set off the day and month of a date within a text.

My birthday makes me feel quite old because I was born on February 16, 1958, in Minnesota.

8. Commas should be used to set up numbers in a text of more than four digits.

We expect 25,000 visitors to the new museum.

QUOTATION MARKS are used for many purposes. First, quotation marks are used to enclose direct quotations within a sentence. Terminal punctuation that is part of the quotation should go inside the marks, and terminal punctuation that is part of the larger sentence goes outside:

She asked him menacingly, "Where is my peanut butter?"

What is the original meaning of the phrase "king of the hill"?

In American English, commas are used to set quotations apart from the following text and are placed inside the marks:

"Although I find him tolerable," Arianna wrote, "I would never want him as a roommate.

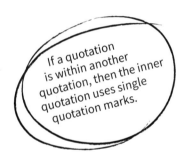
If a quotation is within another quotation, then the inner quotation uses single quotation marks.

Additionally, quotation marks enclose titles of short, or relatively short, literary works such as short stories, chapters, and poems. (The titles of longer works, like novels and anthologies, are italicized.) Writers also use quotation marks to set off words used in special sense or for a non-literary purpose:

The shady dealings of his Ponzi scheme earned him the ironic name "Honest Abe."

APOSTROPHES, sometimes referred to as single quotation marks, show possession; replace missing letters, numerals, and signs; and form plurals of letters, numerals, and signs in certain instances.

1. To signify possession by a singular noun not ending in *s*, add *'s*. (boy → boy's)

2. To signify possession by a singular noun ending in *s*, add *'s*. (class → class's)

3. To signify possession by an indefinite pronoun not ending in *s*, add *'s*. (someone → someone's)

4. To signify possession by a plural noun not ending in *s*, add *'s*. (children → children's)

5. To signify possession by a plural noun ending in *s*, add only the apostrophe. (boys → boys')

6. To signify possession by singular, compound words

and phrases, add *'s* to the last word in the phrase. (everybody else → everybody else's)

7. To signify joint possession, add *'s* only to the last noun. (John and Mary's house)

8. To signify individual possession, add *'s* to each noun. (John's and Mary's houses)

9. To signify missing letters in a contraction, place the apostrophe where the letters are missing. (do not → don't)

10. To signify missing numerals, place the apostrophe where the numerals are missing. (1989 → '89)

11. There are differing schools of thought regarding the pluralization of numerals and dates, but be consistent within the document with whichever method you choose. (1990's/1990s) (A's/As)

Other marks of punctuation include:

- EN DASH (–): to indicate a range of dates
- EM DASH (—): to indicate an abrupt break in a sentence and emphasize the words within the em dashes
- PARENTHESES ( ): to enclose insignificant information
- BRACKETS [ ]: to enclose added words to a quotation and to add insignificant information within parentheses
- SLASH (/): to separate lines of poetry within a text or to indicate interchangeable terminology
- ELLIPSES (…): to indicate information removed from a quotation, to indicate a missing line of poetry, or to create a reflective pause

EXAMPLES

1. Identify the marks of punctuation needed in the following sentence:

   Freds brother wanted the following items for Christmas a red car a condo and a puppy.

   A) Fred's / Christmas; / car, /condo,

   B) Fred's / Christmas: / car, / condo,

   C) Fred's / Christmas: / red, / car,

   D) Fred's / items' / Christmas: / car, / condo,

   B) is correct. To be possessive, *Fred's* requires an apostrophe before the *s*. *Christmas* needs a colon to indicate the upcoming list, and *car* and *condo* should be followed by commas since they are items in a series.

Avoiding Common Usage Errors

Errors in Agreement

Some of the most common grammatical errors are those involving agreement between subjects and verbs, and between nouns and pronouns. While it is impossible to cover all possible errors, the lists below include the most common agreement rules to look for on the test.

SUBJECT/VERB AGREEMENT

1. Single subjects agree with single verbs; plural subjects agree with plural verbs.

    The <u>girl walks</u> her dog.

    The <u>girls walk</u> their dogs.

2. Compound subjects joined by *and* typically take a plural verb unless considered one item.

    <u>Correctness and precision are required</u> for all good writing.

    <u>Macaroni and cheese makes</u> a great snack for children.

3. Compound subjects joined by *or* or *nor* agree with the nearer or nearest subject.

    Neither <u>I nor my friends are</u> looking forward to our final exams.

    Neither <u>my friends nor I am</u> looking forward to our final exams.

4. For sentences with inverted word order, the verb will agree with the subject that follows it.

    Where <u>are Bob and his friends going</u>? Where <u>is Bob going</u>?

> Ignore words between the subject and the verb to help make conjugation clearer:
> The new <u>library</u> ~~with its many books and rooms~~ <u>fills</u> a long-felt need.

5. All single, indefinite pronouns agree with single verbs.
   <u>Neither</u> of the students <u>is</u> happy about the play.
   <u>Each</u> of the many cars <u>is</u> on the grass.
   Every <u>one</u> of the administrators <u>speaks</u> highly of Trevor.

6. All plural, indefinite pronouns agree with plural verbs.
   <u>Several</u> of the students <u>are</u> happy about the play.
   <u>Both</u> of the cars <u>are</u> on the grass.
   <u>Many</u> of the administrators <u>speak</u> highly of Trevor.

7. Collective nouns agree with singular verbs when the collective acts as one unit. Collective nouns agree with plural verbs when the collective acts as individuals within the group.
   The <u>band plans</u> a party after the final football game.
   The <u>band play</u> their instruments even if it rains.
   The <u>jury announces</u> its decision after sequestration.
   The <u>jury make</u> phone calls during their break time.

8. The linking verbs agree with the subject and the predicate.
   My <u>favorite is</u> strawberries and apples.
   My <u>favorites are</u> strawberries and apples.

9. Nouns that are plural in form but singular in meaning will agree with singular verbs.
   <u>Measles is</u> a painful disease.
   <u>Sixty dollars is</u> too much to pay for that book.

10. Singular verbs come after titles, business corporations, and words used as terms.
    <u>"Three Little Kittens" is</u> a favorite nursery rhyme for many children.
    <u>General Motors is</u> a major employer for the city.

PRONOUN/ANTECEDENT AGREEMENT

1. Antecedents joined by *and* typically require a plural pronoun.
   The <u>children and their dogs</u> enjoyed <u>their</u> day at the beach.

2. For compound antecedents joined by *or*, the pronoun agrees with the nearer or nearest antecedent.
   Either the resident mice <u>or the manager's cat</u> gets <u>itself</u> a meal of good leftovers.

3. When indefinite pronouns function in a sentence, the pronoun must agree with the number of the pronoun.

Neither student finished his or her assignment.

Both of the students finished their assignments.

4. When collective nouns function as antecedents, the pronoun choice will be singular or plural depending on the function of the collective.

The audience was cheering as it rose to its feet in unison.

Our family are spending their vacations in Maine, Hawaii, and Rome.

5. When *each* and *every* precede the antecedent, the pronoun agreement will be singular.

Each and every man, woman, and child brings unique qualities to his or her family.

Every creative writer, technical writer, and research writer is attending his or her assigned lecture.

Errors in Sentence Construction

ERRORS IN PARALLELISM occur when items in a series are not put in the same form. For example, if a list contains two nouns and a verb, the sentence should be rewritten so that all three items are the same part of speech. Parallelism should be maintained in words, phrases, and clauses:

The walls were painted green and gold.

Her home is up the hill and beyond the trees.

If we shop on Friday and if we have enough time, we will then visit the aquarium.

SENTENCE ERRORS fall into three categories: fragments, comma splices (comma fault), and fused sentences (run-on). A FRAGMENT occurs when a group of words does not have both a subject and verb as needed to construct a complete sentence or thought. Many times a writer will mirror conversation and write down only a dependent clause, for example, which will have a subject and verb but will not have a complete thought grammatically.

Incorrect. Why are you not going to the mall? Because I do not like shopping.

Correct. Because I do not like shopping, I will not plan to go to the mall.

A COMMA SPLICE (comma fault) occurs when two independent clauses are joined together with only a comma to "splice" them together. To fix a comma splice, a coordinating conjunction should be added, or the comma can be replaced by a semi-colon:

Incorrect. My family eats turkey at Thanksgiving, we eat ham at Christmas.

Correct. My family eats turkey at Thanksgiving, and we eat ham at Christmas.

Correct. My family eats turkey at Thanksgiving; we eat ham at Christmas.

FUSED (run-on) sentences occur when two independent clauses are joined with no punctuation whatsoever. Like comma splices, they can be fixed with a comma and conjunction or with a semi-colon:

Incorrect. My sister lives nearby she never comes to visit.

Correct. My sister lives nearby, but she never comes to visit.

Correct. My sister lives nearby; she never comes to visit.

Commonly Confused Words

a, an: *a* is used before words beginning with consonants or consonant sounds; *an* is used before words beginning with vowels or vowel sounds.

affect, effect: *affect* is most often a verb; *effect* is usually a noun. (*The experience affected me significantly* OR *The experience had a significant effect on me.*)

among, amongst, between: *among* is used for a group of more than two people; *amongst* is archaic and not commonly used in modern writing; *between* is reserved to distinguish two people, places, things, or groups.

amount, number: *amount* is used for non-countable sums; *number* is used with countable nouns. (*She had a large amount of money in her purse, nearly fifty dollars.*)

cite, site: *cite* is a verb used in documentation to credit an author of a quotation, paraphrase, or summary; *site* is a location.

elicit, illicit: *elicit* means to draw out a response from an audience or a listener; *illicit* refers to illegal activity.

every day, everyday: *every day* is an indefinite adjective modifying a noun—*each day* could be used interchangeably with *every day*; *everyday* is a one-word adjective to imply frequent occurrence.

(*Our visit to the Minnesota State Fair is an everyday activity during August.*)

fewer, less: *fewer* is used with a countable noun; *less* is used with a non-countable noun. (*Fewer parents are experiencing stress since the new teacher was hired; parents are experiencing less stress since the new teacher was hired.*)

firstly, secondly: These words are archaic; today, *first* and *second* are more commonly used.

good, well: *good* is always the adjective; *well* is always the adverb except in cases of health. (*She felt well after the surgery.*)

implied, inferred: *implied* is something a speaker does; *inferred* is something the listener does after assessing the speaker's message. (*The speaker implied something mysterious, but I inferred the wrong thing.*)

irregardless, regardless: *irregardless* is non-standard usage and should be avoided; *regardless* is the proper usage of the transitional statement.

its, it's: *its* is a possessive case pronoun; *it's* is a contraction for *it is*.

moral, morale: *moral* is a summative lesson from a story or life event; *morale* is the emotional attitude of a person or group of people.

principal, principle: *principal* is the leader of a school in the noun usage; *principal* means *main* in the adjectival usage; *principle* is a noun meaning *idea* or *tenet*. (*The principal of the school spoke on the principal meaning of the main principles of the school.*)

quote, quotation: *quote* is a verb and should be used as a verb; *quotation* is the noun and should be used as a noun.

reason why: *reason why* is a redundant expression—use one or the other. (*The reason we left is a secret. Why we left is a secret.*)

should of, should have: *should of* is improper usage, likely resulting from misunderstood speech—*of* is not a helping verb and can therefore cannot complete the verb phrase; *should have* is the proper usage. (*He should have driven.*)

than, then: *than* sets up a comparison of some kind; *then* indicates a reference to a point in time. (*When I said that I liked the hat better than the gloves, my sister laughed; then she bought both for me.)

their, there, they're: *their* is the possessive case of the pronoun *they*. *There* is the demonstrative pronoun indicating location, or place. *They're* is a contraction of the words *they are*, the third-person plural subject pronoun and third-person plural, present-tense conjugation of the verb *to be*. These words are very commonly confused in written English.

to lie (to recline), to lay (to place): *to lie* is the intransitive verb meaning *to recline*, so the verb does not take an object; *to lay* is the transitive verb meaning *to place something*. (*I lie out in the sun; I lay my towel on the beach.*)

to try and: *to try and* is sometimes used erroneously in place of *to try to*. (*She should try to succeed daily.*)

unique: *unique* is an ultimate superlative. The word *unique* should not be modified technically. (*The experience was ~~very~~ unique.*)

who, whom: *who* is the subject relative pronoun. (*My son, who is a good student, studies hard.*) Here, the son is carrying out the action of studying, so the pronoun is a subject pronoun (*who*). *Whom* is the object relative pronoun. (*My son, whom the other students admire, studies hard.*) Here, *son* is the object of the other students' admiration, so the pronoun standing in for him, *whom*, is an object pronoun.

your, you're: *your* is the possessive case of the pronoun *you*. *You're* is a contraction of the words *you are*, the second-person subject pronoun and the second-person singular, present-tense conjugation of the verb *to be*. These words are commonly confused in written English.

EXAMPLES

1. Which sentence does NOT contain an error?
    A) My sister and my best friend lives in Chicago.
    B) My parents or my brother is going to pick me up from the airport.
    C) Neither of the students refuse to take the exam.
    D) The team were playing a great game until the rain started.

B) is correct. The verb agrees with the closest subject—in this case, the singular *brother*.

2. Which sentence does NOT contain an error?

   A) The grandchildren and their cousins enjoyed their day at the beach.

   B) Most of the grass has lost their deep color.

   C) The jury was cheering as their commitment came to a close.

   D) Every boy and girl must learn to behave themselves in school.

   A) is correct. *Grandchildren and cousins/their*

3. Which of the following sentence errors is labeled correctly?

   A) Since she went to the store. (fused)

   B) The football game ended in a tie, the underdog caught up in the fourth quarter. (fragment)

   C) The football game ended in a tie the underdog caught up in the fourth quarter. (fused)

   D) When the players dropped their gloves, a fight broke out on the ice hockey rink floor. (comma splice)

   C) is correct. These two independent clauses in C) are fused because there is no punctuation where the two clauses meet.

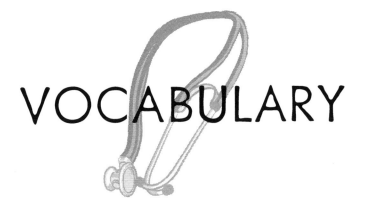

eleven

VOCABULARY

Like the Reading test, the English portion of the TEAS will ask you to identify the meaning of certain words. These words will only appear in a single sentence, not in a passage, so you'll have minimal context clues. Instead, you'll need to learn how to use the word itself to find the meaning. You'll also be asked about the common rules of spelling.

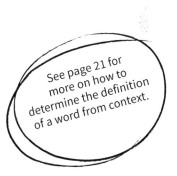

See page 21 for more on how to determine the definition of a word from context.

Word Structure

In addition to using the context of the sentence and passage to determine the meaning of an unfamiliar word, the word itself can give you clues about its meaning. Each word consists of distinct pieces that help determine meaning; the most familiar of these pieces are root words, prefixes, and suffixes.

Root Words

ROOT WORDS are bases from which many words take their foundational form and meaning. The most common root words are Greek and Latin, and a broad knowledge of these roots can greatly improve your ability to determine the meaning of words in context. Knowing root words cannot always provide the exact meaning of a word, but combined with an understanding of the word's place in the sentence and the context surrounding the word, it will often be enough to answer a question about meaning or relationships.

Table 11.1. List of Common Roots

Roots	Meaning	Examples
alter	other	alternate, alter ego
ambi	both	ambidextrous
ami, amic	love	amiable
amphi	both ends or all sides	amphibian

anthrop	man, human, humanity	misanthrope, anthropologist
apert	open	aperture
aqua	water	aqueduct, aquarium
aud	to hear	audience
auto	self	autobiography
bell	war	belligerent, bellicose
bene	good	benevolent
bio	life	biology
ced	yield, go	secede, intercede
cent	one hundred	century
chron	time	chronological
circum	around	circumference
contra/counter	against	contradict
crac, crat	rule, ruler	autocrat, bureacrat
crypt	hidden	cryptogram, cryptic
curr, curs, cours	to run	precursory
dict	to say	dictator, dictation
dyna	power	dynamic
dys	bad, hard, unlucky	dysfunctional
equ	equal, even	equanimity
fac	to make, to do	factory
form	shape	reform, conform
fort	strength	fortitude
fract	to break	fracture
grad, gress	step	progression
gram	thing written	epigram
graph	writing	graphic
hetero	different	heterogeneous
homo	same	homogenous
hypo	below, beneath	hypothermia
iso	identical	isolate
ject	throw	projection
logy	study of	biology
luc	light	elucidate
mal	bad	malevolent
meta, met	behind, between	metacognition- behind the thinking
meter/metr	measure	thermometer
micro	small	microbe
mis/miso	hate	misanthrope
mit	to send	transmit
mono	one	monologue
morph	form, shape	morphology
mort	death	mortal

multi	many	multiple
phil	love	philanthropist
port	carry	transportation
pseudo	false	pseudonym
psycho	soul, spirit	psychic
rupt	to break	disruption
scope	viewing instrument	microscope
scrib/scribe	to write	inscription
sect/sec	to cut	section
sequ, secu	follow	consecutive
soph	wisdom, knowledge	philosophy
spect	to look	spectator
struct	to build	restructure
tele	far off	telephone
terr	earth	terrestrial
therm	heat	thermal
ven, vent	to come	convene
vert	turn	vertigo
voc	voice, call	vocalize, evocative

Prefixes

In addition to understanding the root of a word, it is vital to recognize common affixes that change the meaning of words and demonstrate their relationships to other words. PREFIXES are added to the beginning of a word and frequently change the meaning of the word itself by indicating an opposite or another specifically altered meaning.

Table 11.2. Examples of Prefixes

PREFIXES	MEANING	EXAMPLES
a, an	without, not	anachronism, anhydrous
ab, abs, a	apart, away from	abscission, abnormal
ad	toward	adhere
agere	act	agent
amphi, ambi	round, both sides	ambivalent
ante	before	antedate, anterior
anti	against	antipathy
archos	leader, first, chief	oligarchy
bi	two	binary, bivalve
bene	well, favorable	benevolent, beneficent
caco	bad	cacophny
circum	around	circumnavigate
corpus	body	corporeal

credo	belief	credible
demos	people	demographic
di	two, double	dimorphism, diatomic
dia	across, through	dialectic
dis	not, apart	disenfranchise
dynasthai	be able	dynamo, dynasty
ego	I, self	egomaniac, egocentric
epi	upon, over	epigram, epiphyte
ex	out	extraneous, extemporaneous
geo	earth	geocentric, geomancy
ideo	idea	ideology, ideation
in	in	induction, indigenous
In, im	not	ignoble, immoral
inter	between	interstellar
lexis	word	lexicography
liber	free, book	liberal
locus	place	locality
macro	large	macrophage
micro	small	micron
mono	one, single	monocle, monovalent
mortis	death	moribund
olig	few	oligarchy
peri	around	peripatetic, perineum
poly	many	polygamy
pre	before	prescient
solus	alone	solitary
subter	under, secret	subterfuge
un	not	unsafe
utilis	useful	utilitarian

Suffixes

A SUFFIX, on the other hand, is added to the end of a word and generally indicates the word's relationship to other words in the sentence. Suffixes can change the part of speech or indicate if a word is plural or related to a plural.

Table 11.3. Examples of Suffixes

SUFFIXES	MEANING	EXAMPLES
able, ible	able, capable	visible
age	act of, state of, result of	wreckage
al	relating to	gradual
algia	pain	myalgia
an, ian	native of, relating to	riparian

Suffix	Meaning	Example
ance, ancy	action, process, state	defiance
ary, ery, ory	relating to, quality, place	aviary
cian	processing a specific skill or art	physician
cule, ling	very small	sapling, animalcule
cy	action, function	normalcy
dom	quality, realm	wisdom
ee	one who receives the action	nominee
en	made of, to make	silken
ence, ency	action, state of, quality	urgency
er, or	one who, that which	professor
escent	in the process of	adolescent, senescence
esis, osis	action, process, condition	genesis, neurosis
et, ette	small one, group	baronet, lorgnette
fic	making, causing	specific
ful	full of	frightful
hood	order, condition, quality	adulthood
ice	condition, state, quality	malice
id, ide	a thing connected with or belonging to	bromide
ile	relating to, suited for, capable of	purile, juvenile
ine	nature of	feminine
ion, sion, tion	act, result, or state of	contagion
ish	origin, nature, resembling	impish
ism	system, manner, condition, characteristic	capitalism
ist	one who, that which	artist, flautist
ite	nature of, quality of, mineral product	graphite
ity, ty	state of, quality	captivity
ive	causing, making	exhaustive
ize, ise	make	idolize, bowdlerize
ment	act of, state or, result	containment
nomy	law	autonomy, taxonomy
oid	resembling	asteroid, anthropoid
some	like, apt, tending to	gruesome
strat	cover	strata
tude	state of, condition of	aptitude
um	forms single nouns	spectrum
ure	state of, act, process, rank	rupture, rapture
ward	in the direction of	backward
y	inclined to, tend to	faulty

EXAMPLES

1. Which of the following prefixes should be added to a word to indicate that something is large?

   A) micro

   B) macro

   C) anti

   D) ante

   B) is correct. The prefix *macro–* means *large*.

2. In the sentence below, the prefix *poly–* and the suffix *–glot* in the word *polyglot* indicate that the writer's sister does which of the following?

   My sister is a <u>polyglot</u>, and comfortably travels all over the world.

   A) speaks many language

   B) loves to travel

   C) finds new jobs easily

   D) is unafraid of new places

   A) is correct. The prefix *poly–* means *many*, and the suffix *–glot* means *in a language or tongue*. Therefore, the writer's sister speaks many languages.

Homophones and Homographs

HOMOPHONES are words that sound the same but have different meanings; HOMOGRAPHS are words that are spelled the same way but have different meanings. On the TEAS, you may be asked to identify which homophone is appropriate in the given context, or you may need to identify the correct definition of a homograph as it is used in a sentence.

A good knowledge of homophones is especially important as many words applicable to medicine (*heel/heal, oral/aural*) may be homophones. Is a patient healing, or does he or she have a heel problem? Should medication be administered orally or aurally? Does the patient have a tic, or has he or she been bitten by a tick?

Examples of homophones include:

- tic/tick
- gait/gate
- mail/male
- pain/pane
- oral/aural
- heel/heal

Examples of homographs include:

- tear (to rip/liquid produced by the eye)
- compound (to mix/an enclosed area that includes a building or group of buildings)
- bank (a place to store money/the side of a river/a stockpile)
- novel (a piece of fiction/something new)
- change (to make different/money left over after a transaction)
- rose (a flower/to move upward)
- die (to pass away/a six-sided, numbered cube)

EXAMPLES

Which of the following is the best synonym for *proceeds* as used in the sentence?

The <u>proceeds</u> from the dance will be donated to a local charity.

A) entertainment

B) movement

C) profit

D) snacks

C) is correct. *Proceeds* **can mean either** *profit* **or** *moving forward.* **In this sentence, it is used to mean** *profit* **because** *profit* **can be donated to charity and thus makes sense in the context of the sentence.**

Spelling

A knowledge of spelling is essential for the TEAS. Homophones, basic rules of spelling, and commonly misspelled words will be tested.

Rules of Spelling

English spelling can be complex and confusing. Fortunately, the TEAS won't test you on the more obscure or uncommon spelling rules. Instead, you'll be asked to identify misspellings related to common conjugation patterns (like pluralization) and identify commonly misspelled words.

PLURALS

There are several ways to make a word plural. Most commonly, add an –*s* to a word:

doctors

hospitals

For words that already end in an *s*, or that end in *–sh, –ch, –x,* and *–z,* add *–es.*

dresses

brushes

branches

boxes

waltzes

Generally, words that end in *y* are made plural by dropping the *y* and adding *–ies.*

baby → babies

nursery → nurseries

surgery → surgeries

Generally, words that end in *f* are made plural by dropping the *f* and adding *–ves.*

shelf → shelves

scarf → scarves

In medicine, many words are derived from Latin. It is important to know their proper plural forms.

vertebra → vertebrae

bronchus → bronchi

I before *E*

The phrase *I before E except after C* or *when sounded like A as in neighbor or weigh* is helpful in order to remember the relationship between the vowels *i* and *e* in words.

bel<u>ie</u>ve

conc<u>ei</u>ve

r<u>ei</u>gn

Change a Final *Y* to *I*

If adding a suffix to a word ending in *y*, the *y* must be changed to an *i*, unless the suffix itself begins with *i* or unless a vowel immediately precedes the final *y* in the root word.

plenty + –ful → plentiful

justify + –ing → justifying

justify + –ed → justified

display + –ed → displayed

Double Final Consonant

When adding a suffix like *–ed* or *–ing* to a word ending in a consonant, that final consonant is usually doubled if it is preceded by one vowel and completes a one-syllable word or accented syllable.

refer + –ed → referred

It's doubled because the consonant ends on an accented syllable (re-FER) and is preceded by *one* vowel (ref<u>e</u>r).

limit + –ing → limiting

It's not doubled because the consonant does not end an accented syllable (LI-mit).

seep + –ed → seeped

It's not doubled because the final *p* is preceded by more than one vowel.

consent + –ed → consented

It's not doubled because the final *t* is not preceded by a vowel.

DROP FINAL *E*

Usually, if a root ends with *e*, the *e* is dropped when adding a suffix unless the suffix begins with a consonant.

measure + ing → measuring

measure + ment → measur<u>e</u>ment

Commonly Misspelled Words

a lot	acceptable
accidentally	accommodate
acknowledgement	acquire
acquit	amateur
analysis	argument
beginning	calendar
category	changeable
column	committed
conceivable	conscientious
consensus	definitely
eighth	embarrassment
equipment	especially
exhilarate	existence
foreign	guarantee
generally	government
harass	humorous
immediate	immediately
inoculate	judgment
leisure	liaison
license	lightning
loneliness	maintenance
maneuver	medieval

millennium	minuscule
mischievous	necessary
neighbor	noticeable
occasionally	parallel
personnel	playwright
possession	proceed
profession	publicly
pursue	questionnaire
quizzes	restaurant
receive	recommend
referred	rhyme
rhythm	schedule
separate	sincerely
supersede	technique
unanimous	vacuum
weird	

EXAMPLES

1. Which of the following is misspelled in the sentence below?

    Respondents were asked to complete a simple questionnaire to determine their eligability.

    A) respondents

    B) questionnaire

    C) determine

    D) eligability

    D) is correct. *Eligability* should be spelled *eligibility*.

2. Which of the following nouns is written in the correct plural form?

    A) monkies

    B) parties

    C) watchs

    D) sheeps

    B) is correct. Only *parties* **has been made plural correctly.**

Capitalization

In the following table, there is a list of common capitalization rules. These rules do not encompass every instance when a word should be capitalized, but the table does offer the most common instances that are likely to appear on the TEAS test.

Table 11.4. Capitalization Rules

RULE	Example
Words that begin sentences should be capitalized.	The vitals of the patient are normal.
Proper nouns, names of people, places (e.g. bodies of water, countries, cities, streets), and things (e.g. buildings, monuments, colleges, brands, companies) should be capitalized.	In order to follow his lifelong dream, Griffin accepted a job as a traveling nurse and moved to Budapest.
Titles should be capitalized when used as a part of a person's name.	Attorney General Kasabian, Governor Maxwell, and Dr. Fischer will all be attending the charity dinner tonight.
Titles of publications, books, movies, songs, works of art, etc. should be capitalized, including all words except for prepositions and conjunctions.	She referred to her textbook list: Fundamentals of Nursing, Anatomy and Physiology in Health and Illness, and The Comfort Garden: Tales from the Trauma Unit.
The pronoun I should always be capitalized.	He and I have never understood one another.

PART V: TEST YOUR KNOWLEDGE

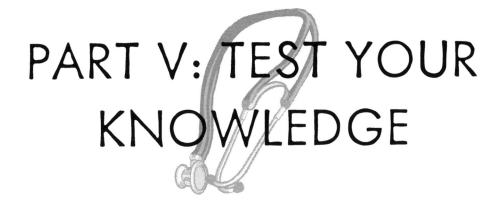

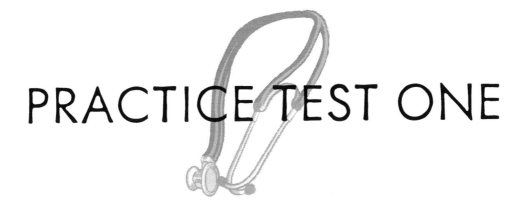

twelve

PRACTICE TEST ONE

Mathematics

Directions: Read the problem carefully, and choose the best answer.

1. A car dealership's commercials claim that this year's models are 20% off the list price, plus they will pay the first 3 monthly payments. If a car is listed for $26,580, and the monthly payments are set at $250, which of the following is the total potential savings?

   A) $1,282
   B) $5,566
   C) $6,066
   D) $20,514

2. A dry cleaner charges $3 per shirt, $6 per pair of pants, and an extra $5 per item for mending. Annie drops off 5 shirts and 4 pairs of pants, 2 of which need mending. Assuming the cleaner charges an 8% sales tax, which of the following will be the amount of Annie's total bill?

   A) $45.08
   B) $49.00
   C) $52.92
   D) $88.20

3. A sandwich shop earns $4 for every sandwich ($s$) it sells, $2 for every drink ($d$), and $1 for every cookie ($c$). If this is all the shop sells, which of the following equations represents what the shop's revenue (r) is over three days?

   A) $r = 4s + 2d + 1c$
   B) $r = 8s + 4d + 2c$
   C) $r = 12s + 6d + 3c$
   D) $r = 16s + 8d + 4c$

4. Which of the following is the y-intercept of the line whose equation is $7y - 42x + 7 = 0$?

   A) $(\frac{1}{6}, 0)$
   B) $(6, 0)$
   C) $(0, -1)$
   D) $(-1, 0)$

5. $4 - \frac{1}{2^2} + 24 \div (8 + 12)$
   Simplify the expression. Which of the following is correct?

   A) 1.39
   B) 2.74
   C) 4.95
   D) 15.28

6. A rectangular field has area of 1452 square feet. If the width is three times greater than the length, which of the following is the length of the field?

   A) 22 feet

   B) 44 feet

   C) 242 feet

   D) 1452 feet

7. The owner of a newspaper has noticed that print subscriptions have gone down 40% while online subscriptions have gone up 60%. Print subscriptions once accounted for 70% of the newspaper's business, and online subscriptions accounted for 25%. Which of the following is the overall percentage growth or decline in business?

   A) 13% decline

   B) 15% decline

   C) 28% growth

   D) Business has stayed the same.

8. $(6.4)(2.8) \div 0.4$

   Simplify the expression. Which of the following is correct?

   A) 16.62

   B) 17.92

   C) 41.55

   D) 44.80

9. Bridget is repainting her rectangular bedroom. Two walls measure 15 feet by 9 feet, and the other two measure 12.5 feet by 9 feet. One gallon of paint covers an average of 32 square meters. Which of the following is the number of gallons of paint that Bridget will use? (There are 3.28 feet in 1 meter.)

   A) 0.72 gallons

   B) 1.43 gallons

   C) 4.72 gallons

   D) 15.5 gallons

10. $5\frac{2}{3} \times 1\frac{7}{8} \div \frac{1}{3}$

    Simplify the expression. Which of the following is correct?

    A. $3\frac{13}{24}$

    B. $6\frac{3}{4}$

    C. $15\frac{3}{4}$

    D. $31\frac{7}{8}$

11. Based on a favorable performance review at work, Matt receives a $\frac{3}{20}$ increase in his hourly wage. If his original hourly wage is represented by w, which of the following represents his new wage?

    A) $0.15w$

    B) $0.85w$

    C) $1.12w$

    D) $1.15w$

12. A restaurant employs servers, hosts, and managers in a ratio of 9:2:1. If there are 36 total employees, which of the following is the number of hosts at the restaurant?

    A) 3

    B) 4

    C) 6

    D) 8

13. If x is the proportion of men who play an instrument, y is the proportion of women who play an instrument, and z is the total number of men, which of the following is true?

    A. $\frac{z}{x}$ = number of men who play an instrument

    B. $(1 - z)x$ = number of men who do not play an instrument

    C. $(1 - x)z$ = number of men who do not play an instrument

    D. $(1 - y)z$ = number of women who do not play an instrument

14. A woman's dinner bill comes to $48.30. If she adds a 20% tip, which of the following will be her total bill?

    A) $9.66

    B) $38.64

    C) $48.30

    D) $57.96

15. Which of the following lists is in order from least to greatest?

    A) $\frac{1}{7}$, 0.125, $\frac{6}{9}$, 0.60

    B) $\frac{1}{7}$, 0.125, 0.60, $\frac{6}{9}$

    C) 0.125, $\frac{1}{7}$, 0.60, $\frac{6}{9}$

    D) 0.125, $\frac{1}{7}$, 0.125, $\frac{6}{9}$, 0.60

16. Which of the following is equivalent to 3.28?

    A) $3\frac{1}{50}$

    B) $3\frac{1}{25}$

    C) $3\frac{7}{50}$

    D) $3\frac{7}{25}$

17. $x \div 7 = x - 36$

    Solve the equation. Which of the following is correct?

    A) $x = 6$

    B) $x = 42$

    C) $x = 126$

    D) $x = 252$

18. After taxes, a worker earned $15,036 in 7 months. Which of the following is the amount the worker earned in 2 months?

    A) $2,148

    B) $4,296

    C) $6,444

    D) $8,592

19. If m represents a car's average mileage in miles per gallon, p represents the price of gas in dollars per gallon, and d represents a distance in miles, which of the following algebraic equations represents the cost c of gas per mile?

    A) $c = \frac{dp}{m}$

    B) $c = \frac{p}{m}$

    C) $c = \frac{mp}{d}$

    D) $c = \frac{m}{p}$

20. Melissa is ordering fencing to enclose a square area of 5625 square feet. Which of the following is the number of feet of fencing she needs?

    A) 75 feet

    B) 150 feet

    C) 300 feet

    D) 5,625 feet

21. Adam is painting the outside of a 4-walled shed. The shed is 5 feet wide, 4 feet deep, and 7 feet high. Which of the following is the amount of paint Adam will need for the four walls?

    A) 80 ft.^{2}

    B) 126 ft.^{2}

    C) 140 ft.^{2}

    D) 560 ft.^{2}

22. A circular swimming pool has a circumference of 49 feet. Which of the following is the diameter of the pool?

    A) 15.6 feet

    B) 17.8 feet

    C) 49 feet

    D) 153.9 feet

23.

Table 12.1. Employee Hours

EMPLOYEE	HOURS WORKED
Suzanne	42
Joe	38
Mark	25
Ellen	50
Jill	45
Rob	46
Nicole	17
Deb	41

The table above shows the number of hours worked by employees during the week. Which of the following is the median number of hours worked per week by the employees?

A) 38

B) 41

C) 42

D) 41.5

24. According to the graph, which of the following was Sam's average monthly income from January through May? (Round to the nearest hundred.)

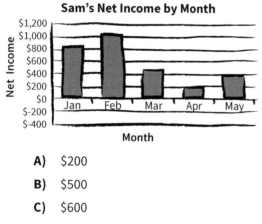

Sam's Net Income by Month

A) $200

B) $500

C) $600

D) $1,100

25. Which of the following is equivalent to 8 pounds and 8 ounces? (Round to the nearest tenth of a kilogram.)

A) 3.6 kilograms

B) 3.9 kilograms

C) 17.6 kilograms

D) 18.7 kilograms

26. $(4.71 \times 10^3) - (2.98 \times 10^2)$

Simplify the expression. Which of the following is correct?

A) 1.73×10

B) 4.412×10^2

C) 1.73×10^3

D) 4.412×10^3

27. Which of the following is not a negative value?

A) $(-3)(-1)(2)(-1)$

B) $14 - 7 + (-7)$

C) $7 - 10 + (-8)$

D) $-5(-2)(-3)$

28. $10^2 - 7(3 - 4) - 25$

Simplify the expression. Which of the following is correct?

A) -12

B) 2

C) 68

D) 82

29. $\dfrac{5^2(3) + 3(-2)^2}{4 + 3^2 - 2(5 - 8)}$

Simplify the expression. Which of the following is correct?

A) $\dfrac{9}{8}$

B) $\dfrac{87}{19}$

C) 9

D) $\dfrac{21}{2}$

30. Anna is buying fruit at the farmers' market. She selects 1.2 kilograms of apples, 800 grams of bananas, and 300 grams of strawberries. The farmer charges her a flat rate of $4 per kilogram. Which of the following is the total cost of her produce?

A) $4.40

B) $5.24

C) $9.20

D) $48.80

31. $\left(1\frac{1}{2}\right)\left(2\frac{2}{3}\right) \div 1\frac{1}{4}$

Simplify the expression. Which of the following is correct?

A) $3\frac{1}{12}$

B) $3\frac{1}{5}$

C) 4

D) 5

32. Which of the following lists is in order from least to greatest?

A) $2^{-1}, -\frac{4}{3}, (-1)^3, \frac{2}{5}$

B) $-\frac{4}{3}, (-1)^3, 2^{-1}, \frac{2}{5}$

C) $-\frac{4}{3}, \frac{2}{5}, 2^{-1}, (-1)^3$

D) $-\frac{4}{3}, (-1)^3, \frac{2}{5}, 2^{-1}$

33. Which of the following is 2.7834 rounded to the nearest tenth?

A) 2.7

B) 2.78

C) 2.8

D) 2.88

34. $\frac{4x-5}{3} = \frac{\frac{1}{2}(2x-6)}{5}$

Simplify the expression. Which of the following is the value of x?

A) $-\frac{2}{7}$

B) $-\frac{4}{17}$

C) $\frac{16}{17}$

D) $\frac{8}{7}$

35. $8x - 6 = 3x + 24$

Solve the equation. Which of the following is correct?

A) $x = 2.5$

B) $x = 3.6$

C) $x = 5$

D) $x = 6$

36. A student gets 42 questions out of 48 correct on a quiz. Which of the following is the percentage of questions that the student answered correctly?

A) 1.14%

B) 82.50%

C) 85.00%

D) 87.50%

Reading

Directions: Read the question, passage, or figure carefully, and choose the best answer.

1. Which of the following best captures the author's purpose?

> The social and political discourse of America continues to be permeated with idealism. An idealistic viewpoint asserts that the ideals of freedom, equality, justice, and human dignity are the truths that Americans must continue to aspire to. Idealists argue that truth is what should be, not necessarily what is. In general, they work to improve things and to make them as close to ideal as possible.

A) to advocate for freedom, equality, justice, and human rights

B) to explain what an idealist believes in

C) to explain what's wrong with social and political discourse in America

D) to persuade readers to believe in certain truths

2. The diagram represents a blood pressure monitor. Which of the following represents the systolic blood pressure reading?

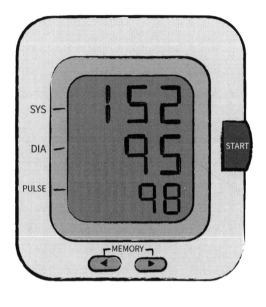

A) 152

B) 95

C) 98

D) $\frac{152}{95}$

The next four questions are based on this passage.

The best friend a man has in the world may turn against him and become his enemy. His son or daughter that he has reared with loving care may prove ungrateful. Those who are nearest and dearest to us, those whom we trust with our happiness and our good name may become traitors to their faith. The money that a man has, he may lose. It flies away from him, perhaps when he needs it most. A man's reputation may be sacrificed in a moment of ill-considered action.

The one absolutely unselfish friend that man can have in this selfish world, the one that never deserts him, the one that never proves ungrateful or treacherous is his dog. A man's dog stands by him in prosperity and in poverty, in health and in sickness. He will sleep on the cold ground, where the wintry winds blow and the snow drives fiercely, if only he may be near his master's side. He will kiss the hand that has no food to offer. He will lick the wounds and sores that come in encounters with the roughness of the world. He guards the sleep of his pauper master as if he were a prince. When all other friends desert, he remains.

George Graham Vest - c. 1855
http://www.historyplace.com/speeches/vest.htm

3. Which of the following best describes the structure of the text?

- **A)** chronology
- **B)** cause and effect
- **C)** problem and solution
- **D)** contrast

4. Which of the following could be considered the topic of this passage?

- **A)** loyal friends
- **B)** misfortune
- **C)** human treachery
- **D)** feeling safe

5. Which of the following is a logical conclusion of the passage?

- **A)** Those closest to you will always betray you.
- **B)** Friendships with other people are pointless.
- **C)** Someone who wants a loyal friend should get a dog.
- **D)** Only a dog can help a person through the rough times in his or her life.

6. Which of the following is the purpose of this passage?

- **A)** to inform
- **B)** to entertain
- **C)** to describe
- **D)** to persuade

The next two questions are based on this passage.

How to Plant Potatoes

Before Planting

Plant potatoes no later than 2 weeks after the last spring freeze.

Cut potatoes into pieces 1 to 2 days before planting.

Loosen soil using a tiller or hand trowel.

Mix fertilizer or compost into loosened soil.

Planting

Dig a 4-inch-deep trench and place potatoes 1 foot apart.

Cover potatoes loosely with soil.

After Planting

Water immediately after planting, and then regularly afterward to keep soil moist.

After 6 weeks, mound soil around the base of the plant to ensure roots stay covered.

7. Which of the following is the first step to take after planting potatoes?

- **A)** Mound soil around the base of the plant.
- **B)** Water immediately.
- **C)** Mix fertilizer or compost into loosened soil.
- **D)** Place potatoes 1 foot apart.

8. Which of the following should be done after the soil has been loosened with a tiller or trowel?

- **A)** Mix fertilizer or compost into loosened soil.
- **B)** Dig a 4-inch-deep trench.
- **C)** Cut potatoes into pieces.
- **D)** Mound soil around the base of the plant.

The next two questions are based on this email.

Alan —

I just wanted to drop you a quick note to let you know I'll be out of the office for the next two weeks. Elizabeth and I are finally taking that trip to France we've been talking about for years. It's a bit of a last-minute decision, but since we had the vacation time available, we figured it was now or never.

Anyway, my team's been briefed on the upcoming meeting, so they should be able to handle the presentation without any hiccups. If you have any questions or concerns, you can direct them to Joanie, who'll be handling my responsibilities while I'm out.

Let me know if you want any special treats. I don't know if you can take chocolate and cheese on the plane, but I'm going to try!

Best regards,

Michael

9. Which of the following most likely describes the relationship between the author and Alan?

A) familial

B) formal

C) friendly

D) strained

10. Which of the following best captures the author's purpose?

A) to ask Alan if he wants any special treats from France

B) to brag to Alan about his upcoming vacation

C) to inform Alan that he will be out of the office

D) to help Alan prepare for the upcoming meeting

The next two questions are based on this map.

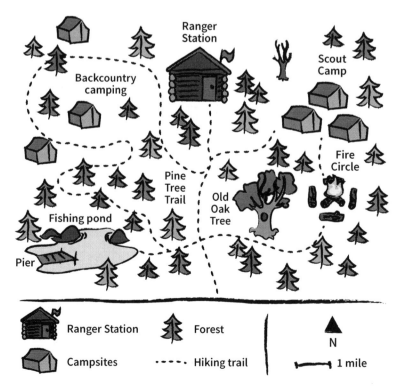

11. Which of the following is located due north of the Fire Circle?

    A) Old Oak Tree

    B) Scout Camp

    C) Fishing Pond

    D) Backcountry Camping

12. If a camper followed the trail from the Fishing Pond to the Scout Camp and passed by the Fire Circle, which of the following would she also have to pass by?

    A) Old Oak Tree

    B) Ranger Station

    C) Backcountry Camping

    D) Pier

The next three questions are based on this passage.

Carl's Car Depot is hosting its one-day-only summer sale event! All sedans, trucks, SUVs, and more are marked to move quickly. We're offering no money down and low (like, really low) monthly payments. You won't find prices like these anywhere else in the city (or the state, or anywhere else you look). No matter what you're looking for, we've the new and used cars you need. We only drop our prices this low once a year, so don't miss out on this great deal!

13. Which of the following best describes the author's purpose?

    A) The author wants to tell customers what kinds of cars are available at Carl's Car Depot.

    B) The author wants to encourage other car dealerships to lower their prices.

    C) The author wants to provide new and used cars at affordable prices.

    D) The author wants to attract customers to Carl's Car Depot.

14. Based on the context, which of the following is the meaning of the word *move* in the passage?

    A) drive

    B) sell

    C) advance forward

    D) change location

15. Which of the following is NOT mentioned by the author as a reason to visit Carl's Car Depot?

    A) They are offering lifetime warranties on new cars.

    B) The sale will only last one day.

    C) They have the lowest prices in town.

    D) They are offering no money down and low monthly payments.

16. Italics are used for which of the following reasons?

> Although Ben *said* he supported for his coworkers, his actions suggested he did not condone their behavior.

    A) to show a word is intentionally misspelled

    B) to indicate a word in a foreign language

    C) to emphasize a contrast

    D) to reference a footnote

The next five questions are based on this passage.

It had been a long morning for Julia. She'd been woken up early by the sound of lawn mowers outside her window, and despite her best efforts, had been unable to get back to sleep. So, she'd reluctantly got out of bed, showered, and prepared her morning cup of coffee. At least, she tried to anyway. In the kitchen she'd discovered she was out of regular coffee and had to settle for a decaffeinated cup instead.

Once on the road, her caffeine-free mug of coffee didn't help make traffic less annoying. In fact, it seemed to Julia like the other drivers were sluggish and surly as well—it took her an extra fifteen minutes to get to work. And when she arrived, all the parking spots were full.

By the time she'd finally found a spot in the overflow lot, she was thirty minutes late for work. She'd hoped her boss would be too busy to notice, but he'd already put a pile of paperwork on her desk with a note that simply said "Rewrite." She wondered if she should point out to her boss that she hadn't been the one to write the reports in the first place, but decided against it.

When the fire alarm went off an hour later, Julia decided she'd had enough. She grabbed her purse and headed outside with her coworkers. While everyone else stood around waiting for the alarm to quiet, Julia determinedly walked to her car, fired up the engine, and set a course for home.

17. Which of the following lists Julia's actions in the correct sequence?

   A) Julia woke up early and found she didn't have any regular coffee. When she got to work, her boss had a lot for her to do. When the fire alarm went off, she decided to go home.

   B) Julia got to work and decided she was too tired to do the work her boss asked for, so she went home to get a cup of coffee.

   C) Julia woke up when the fire alarm went off and couldn't get back to sleep. She then got stuck in traffic and arrived at work thirty minutes late.

   D) Julia was woken up early by a lawnmower and then got stuck in traffic on the way to her office. Once there, she found that the office was out of coffee and she had a lot of work to do. When the fire alarm went off, she decided to go home.

18. Which of the following is the most likely reason Julia did not return to work after the alarm?

   A) She was embarrassed that should could not finish the work her boss asked for.

   B) She was tired and wanted to go home.

   C) She got stuck in traffic and could not get back to her office.

   D) Her boss gave her the afternoon off.

19. Which of the following statements based on the passage should be considered an opinion?

   A) Julia's boss asked her to do work to help one of her coworkers.

   B) Julia was late to work because of traffic.

   C) It was irresponsible for Julia to leave work early.

   D) Julia was tired because she'd been woken up early.

20. The passage states that Julia *set a course for home*. Which of the following is the most accurate interpretation of this sentence?

A) Julia is looking up directions to her house.

B) Julia is planning to drive home.

C) Julia wants to go home but will go back to work.

D) Julia is worried the fire at her office will spread to her home.

21. Which of the following conclusions is best supported by the passage?

A) Julia will find a job closer to her home.

B) Julia will be fired.

C) Julia will feel guilty and return to work.

D) Julia will drive home and go to sleep.

22. In the context of the passage below, which of the following would most likely NOT support a strong federal government?

Alexander Hamilton and James Madison called for the Constitutional Convention to write a constitution as the foundation of a stronger federal government. Madison and other Federalists like John Adams believed in separation of powers, republicanism, and a strong federal government. Despite the separation of powers that would be provided for in the US Constitution, anti-Federalists like Thomas Jefferson called for even more limitations on the power of the federal government.

A) Alexander Hamilton

B) James Madison

C) John Adams

D) Thomas Jefferson

23. Based on the pattern in the headings, which of the following is a reasonable heading to insert in the blank spot?

Chapter 2: Amphibians of Texas

1. Frogs
   A) Tree Frogs
   B) _____
   C) True Frogs

2. Toads
   A) True Toads
   B) Narrowmouth Toads
   C) Burrowing Toads

3. Salamanders

A) Gray Tree Frog

B) Tropical Frogs

C) Newts

D) Spadefoot Toads

24. Which of the following is an example of a secondary source that would be used in a documentary about World War I?

A) an essay by a historian about the lasting effects of the war

B) photographs of military equipment used in the war

C) a recorded interview with a veteran who fought for the US Army

D) letters written by soldiers to their families

25. Based on the context, which of the following is the meaning of the word *match* in the sentence?

Victoria won easily and had plenty of time to rest before her next scheduled match.

A) a competitive event

B) a suitable pair

C) a slender piece of wood used to start a fire

D) a prospective marriage partner

The next two questions are based on this table.

Table 12.2. Book Sales by Distributor

DISTRIBUTOR	COST STRUCTURE
Wholesale Books	$100 for the first 25 books; $80 for every 25 additional books
The Book Barn	$98 for every 25 books
Books and More	$3.99 per book
Quarter Price Books	$3.99 per book for the first 25 books; $2.99 for each additional book

26. A school wants to buy seventy-five textbooks. Based on the pricing chart, which of the following distributors would offer the cheapest price for the books?

   A) Wholesale Books

   B) The Book Barn

   C) Books and More

   D) Quarter Price Books

27. A teacher wants to buy an additional twenty-five books for her classroom. If she orders her books separately, which distributor would offer the cheapest price?

   A) Wholesale Books

   B) The Book Barn

   C) Books and More

   D) Quarter Price Books

The next two questions are based on this passage.

The study showed that private tutoring is providing a significant advantage to those students who are able to afford it. Researchers looked at the grades of students who had received free tutoring through the school versus those whose parents had paid for private tutors. The study included 2500 students in three high schools across four grade levels. The study found that private tutoring corresponded with a rise in grade point average (GPA) of 0.5 compared to students who used the school's free tutor service and 0.7 compared to students who used no tutoring. After reviewing the study, the board is recommending that the school restructure its free tutor service to provide a more equitable education for all students.

28. Which of the following would weaken the author's argument?

   A) the fact that the cited study was funded by a company that provides discounted tutoring through schools

   B) a study showing differences in standardized test scores between students at schools in different neighborhoods

   C) a statement signed by local teachers stating that they do not provide preferential treatment in the classroom or when grading

   D) a study showing that GPA does not strongly correlate with success in college

29. Which of the following types of arguments is used in the passage?

   A) emotional argument

   B) appeal to authority

   C) specific evidence

   D) rhetorical questioning

30. Start with the shapes shown below. Follow the directions.

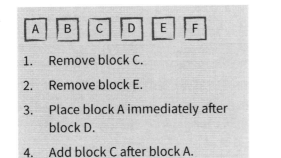

1. Remove block C.
2. Remove block E.
3. Place block A immediately after block D.
4. Add block C after block A.

Which of the following shows the order in which the shapes now appear?

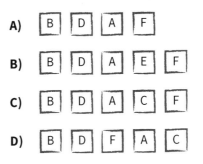

A)

B)

C)

D)

The next two questions are based on this passage.

After looking at five houses, Robert and I have decided to buy the one on Forest Road. The first two homes we visited didn't have the space we need—the first had only one bathroom, and the second did not have a guest bedroom. The third house, on Pine Street, had enough space inside but didn't have a big enough yard for our three dogs. The fourth house we looked at, on Rice Avenue, was stunning but well above our price range. The last home, on Forest Road, wasn't in the neighborhood we wanted to live in. However, it had the right amount of space for the right price.

31. Which of the following lists the author's actions in the correct sequence?

A) The author looked at the house on Forest Road, then at a house with a yard that was too small, then at two houses that were too small, and then finally at a house that was too expensive.

B) The author looked at the house on Forest Road, then at two houses that were too small, then at a house with a yard that was too small, and then finally at a house that was too expensive.

C) The author looked at two homes with yards that were too small, then a house with only one bathroom, then a house that was too expensive, and then finally the house on Forest Road.

D) The author looked at two homes that were too small, then a house with a yard that was too small, then a house that was too expensive, and then finally at the house on Forest Road.

32. What is the author's conclusion about the house on Pine Street?

A) The house did not have enough bedrooms.

B) The house did not have a big enough yard.

C) The house was not in the right neighborhood.

D) The house was too expensive.

33. A student wants to find unbiased information on an upcoming state senate election for a class project. Which of the following sources should the student use?

A) a website run by a candidate's campaign advisor

B) an endorsement of a candidate from a local newspaper

C) a blog run by a local radio personality

D) a book on the history of elections

The next two questions are based on this passage.

Mr. Tim Morgan —

This letter is to inform Mr. Morgan that his application for the position of Lead Technician has been received by our Human Resources team. We have been pleased to receive a higher-than-expected number of applications for this position, and we are glad that Mr. Morgan is among the many who find our company an attractive place to build a career. Due to the influx of applications, our Human Resources team will be taking longer than previously stated to review candidates and schedule interviews. Please look for further communication from our Human Resources team in the next two to three weeks.

Regards,

Allison Wakefield
Head of Human Resources

34. Which of the following best describes the purpose of the passage?

    A) to let Mr. Morgan know that he will likely not receive an offer for the job of Lead Technician due to the high number of applicants

    B) to express to Mr. Morgan how pleased the Human Resources team was to receive his application

    C) to offer Mr. Morgan the position of Lead Technician

    D) to inform Mr. Morgan that the review of candidates will take longer than expected

35. Which of the following conclusions is well supported by the passage?

    A) The Human Resources team had previously informed Mr. Morgan that he would receive feedback on his application in less than two weeks.

    B) Mr. Morgan is well qualified for the position of Lead Technician and will be offered an interview.

    C) The Human Resources team will have trouble finding a qualified candidate for the position of Lead Technician.

    D) Mr. Morgan will respond to this communication by removing himself from consideration for the positon of Lead Technician.

The next three questions are based on this passage.

The greatest changes in sensory, motor, and perceptual development happen in the first two years of life. When babies are first born, most of their senses operate in a similar way to those of adults. For example, babies are able to hear before they are born; studies show that babies turn toward the sound of their mothers' voices just minutes after being born, indicating they recognize the mother's voice from their time in the womb.

The exception to this rule is vision. A baby's vision changes significantly in its first year of life; initially it has a range of vision of only 8 – 12 inches and no depth perception. As a result, infants rely primarily on hearing; vision does not become the dominant sense until around the age of 12 months. Babies also prefer faces to other objects. This preference, along with their limited vision range, means that their sight is initially focused on their caregiver.

36. Which of the following is a concise summary of the passage?

    A) Babies have no depth perception until 12 months, which is why they focus only on their caregivers' faces.

    B) Babies can recognize their mothers' voices when born, so they initially rely primarily on their sense of hearing.

    C) Babies have senses similar to those of adults except for their sense of sight, which doesn't fully develop until 12 months.

    D) Babies' senses go through many changes in the first year of their lives.

37. Which of the following senses do babies primarily rely on?

    A) vision

    B) hearing

    C) touch

    D) smell

38. Which of the following best describes the mode of the passage?

    A) expository

    B) narrative

    C) persuasive

    D) descriptive

39. According to the guide, in which of the following seasons would ginger be harvested?

> **Spring:** artichokes, broccoli, chives, collard greens, peas, spinach, watercress

> **Summer:** beets, bell peppers, corn, eggplant, green beans, okra, tomatoes, zucchini

> **Fall:** acorn squash, brussels sprouts, cauliflower, endive, ginger, sweet potatoes

> **Winter:** Belgian endive, buttercup squash, kale, leeks, turnips, winter squash

    A) spring

    B) summer

    C) fall

    D) winter

The next two questions are based on this passage.

In Greek mythology, two gods, Epimetheus and Prometheus, were given the work of creating living things. Epimetheus gave good powers to the different animals. To the lion he gave strength; to the bird, swiftness; to the fox, sagacity; and so on. Eventually, all of the good gifts had been bestowed, and there was nothing left for humans. As a result, Prometheus returned to heaven and brought down fire, which he gave to humans. With fire, human beings could protect themselves by making weapons. Over time, humans developed civilization.

40. Which of the following is the meaning of the word *bestowed* as it is used in the passage?

    A) purchased

    B) forgotten

    C) accepted

    D) given

41. Which of the following provides the best summary of the passage?

    A) Epimetheus was asked to assign all the good traits to the animals, which upset Prometheus. In retaliation, Prometheus brought fire to humans, which allowed them to reign over the other animals.

B) Epimetheus and Prometheus were both asked to create living things and assign traits to living creatures. Epimetheus gave all of the positive traits to the other animals and left nothing for humans, so Prometheus brought humans fire. This fire allowed human beings to thrive.

C) Epimetheus and Prometheus were given the job of assigning traits to the animals. They decided to give strength to lions, swiftness to birds, sagacity to the fox, and fire to humans. This fire has helped humans grow to be superior to other animals.

D) Prometheus decided that humans needed fire to protect themselves from the other animals. He brought fire down from Heaven and taught humans how to make weapons, which allowed humans to hunt animals.

42. Based on the pattern in the headings, which of the following is a reasonable heading to insert in the blank spot?

3. Balanced Nutrition
   A. Sources of Iron
      1) Animal-Based Sources
        a. Beef
        b. Pork
        c. _____
      2) Plant-Based Sources
        a. Leafy Greens
        b. Nuts and Seeds
   B. Sources of Calcium
   C. Sources of Omega-3 Fatty Acids

A) Dairy

B) Lamb

C) Legumes

D) Vitamins

The next two questions are based on this excerpt.

Table of Contents

1. Renaissance Art...15 – 104
   A) Italian Painters.. 18 – 57
   B) German Painters.. 59 – 72
   C) French Painters.. 73 – 104

2. Renaissance Architecture...105 – 203
   A) Renaissance: 1400 – 1500.. 107 – 152
   B) High Renaissance: 1500 – 1525 .... 153 – 177
   C) Mannerism: 1520 – 1600.. 179 – 203

43. A student wants to find information on the Italian painter Sandro Botticelli. On which of the following pages will the student most likely find this information?

A) 55

B) 71

C) 95

D) 114

44. A student wants to find information on a church built in 1518. On which of the following pages should the student begin to look for this information?

A) 59

B) 105

C) 153

D) 179

The next two questions are based on this passage.

The odds of success for any new restaurant are slim. Competition in the city is fierce, and the low margin of return means that aspiring restaurateurs must be exact and ruthless with their budget and pricing. The fact that The Hot Dog has lasted as long as it has is a testament to its owners' skills.

45. Which of the following conclusions is well supported by the passage?

    A) The Hot Dog offers the best casual dining in town.

    B) The Hot Dog has a well-managed budget and prices items on its menu appropriately.

    C) The popularity of The Hot Dog will likely fall as new restaurants open in the city.

    D) The Hot Dog has a larger margin of return than other restaurants in the city.

46. Which of the following is the meaning of *testament* as used in the sentence?

    A) story

    B) surprise

    C) artifact

    D) evidence

The next two questions are based on this passage.

As you can see from the graph, my babysitting business has been really successful. The year started with a busy couple of months—several snows combined with a large number of requests for Valentine's Day services boosted our sales quite a bit. The spring months have admittedly been a bit slow, but we're hoping for a big summer once school gets out. Several clients have already put in requests for our services!

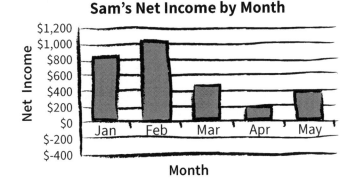

Sam's Net Income by Month

47. Based on the information in the graph, how much more did Sam's Babysitting Service bring in during February than during April?

    A) $200

    B) $900

    C) $1100

    D) $1300

48. Which of the following best describes the tone of the passage?

    A) professional

    B) casual

    C) concerned

    D) neutral

49. The diagram represents the lock and key model of enzymes. According to the figure, the products are formed from which of the following?

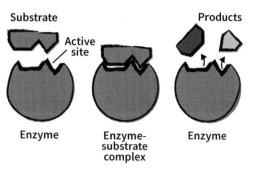

Substrate — Active site — Products

Enzyme — Enzyme-substrate complex — Enzyme

A) the enzyme

B) the enzyme-substrate complex

C) the substrate

D) the active site

50. Which of the following sentences indicates the end of a sequence?

A) Our ultimate objective was to find a quality coat at an affordable price.

B) We chose this particular restaurant because of its outdoor seating.

C) Finally, we were able to settle in to enjoy the movie.

D) Initially, it seemed unlikely that we'd be able to keep the puppy.

51. A student wants to find information on the Battle of the Scheldt. According to the index for a history textbook, where should the student look?

Battle of San Marino	112 – 3, 201
Battle of Sedan	113, 202
Battle of Sidi Barrani	115 – 6
Battle of Someri	203 – 205
Battle of Stalingrad	306 – 310
Battle of Studzianki	307 – 308
Battle of the Scheldt	110 – 2, 207

A) 110

B) 115

C) 203

D) 307

Science

Directions: Read the question carefully, and choose the best answer.

1. Which of the following describes the primary function of the respiratory system?

   A) to create sound and speech

   B) to take oxygen into the body while removing carbon dioxide

   C) to transport nutrients to the cells and tissue of the body

   D) to act as a barrier between the body's organs and outside influences

2. Which of the following is the first step of the scientific method?

   A) construct a hypothesis

   B) make observations

   C) analyze data

   D) form a question

3. The process of organisms with an advantageous trait surviving more often and producing more offspring than organisms without the advantageous trait describes which of the following basic mechanisms of evolution?

   A) gene flow

   B) genetic drift

   C) mutation

   D) natural selection

4. Which of the following is the group of basophils that produces follicle-stimulating hormone (FSH) and luteinizing hormone (LH)?

   A) gonadotrophs

   B) thyrotroph

   C) chromophil

   D) pituicytes

5. Which of the following are considered the basic units of the female reproductive system, each containing a single immature egg cell that is released during ovulation?

   A) oocytes

   B) follicles

   C) ovaries

   D) fundus

6. Which of the following describes the muscular organ that processes food material into increasingly smaller pieces, mixes it with saliva to create a bolus, and creates a barrier to transport food into the esophagus?

   A) pharynx

   B) tongue

   C) diaphragm

   D) stomach

7. Which of the following chambers of the heart receives blood returning from the lungs during pulmonary circulation?

   A) left atrium

   B) right atrium

   C) left ventricle

   D) right ventricle

8. Which of the following is the lobe in the cerebral cortex primarily responsible for processing and integrating sensory information received from the rest of the body?

   A) frontal lobe

   B) occipital lobe

   C) parietal lobe

   D) temporal lobe

9. Which of the following is an example of adaptive, or specific, immunity?

A) inflammation

B) fever

C) humoral

D) phagocytosis

10. Which of the following describes a situation in which research results are consistent with every subsequent experiment, but the test used in the experiment does not measure what it claims to measure?

A) reliable, but not valid

B) valid, but not reliable

C) neither reliable nor valid

D) both reliable and valid

11. Which of the following Mendellian laws describes how pairs of alleles within genes separate and recombine separately from other genes?

A) law of segregation

B) law of dominance

C) law of independent assortment

D) law of predictive traits

12. Which of the following describes how atomic radius varies across the periodic table?

A) Atomic radius increases from top to bottom and left to right on the periodic table.

B) Atomic radius increases from top to bottom and right to left on the periodic table.

C) Atomic radius increases from top to bottom and toward the halogens on the periodic table.

D) Atomic radius increases from top to bottom and toward the noble gases on the periodic table.

13. Which of the following is NOT a tissue layer found in skeletal bone?

A) periosteum

B) bone marrow

C) enamel

D) cancellous bone

14. Which of the following sets of valves is primarily responsible for preventing blood flow from major blood vessels to the heart?

A) atrioventricular valves

B) semilunar valves

C) tricuspid valves

D) bicuspid valves

15. Which of the following is the connective area where nerve impulses send neurotransmitters across a synapse to a muscle cell to stimulate muscle contraction?

A) sarcomere

B) tendon

C) nicotinic receptors

D) neuromuscular junction

16. Bone is composed primarily of which of the following inorganic materials?

A) calcium

B) magnesium

C) collagen

D) potassium

17. Which of the following is the region of the brain that controls and regulates autonomic functions such as respiration, digestion, and heart rate?

A) cerebellum

B) medulla oblongata

C) temporal lobe

D) cerebral cortex

18. Which of the following is the primary physical barrier the body uses to prevent infection?

   A) mucus membranes

   B) stomach acid

   C) skin

   D) urine

19. Which of the following describes the primary function of the pyloric sphincter?

   A) to regulate the movement of digested food material from the stomach to the duodenum

   B) to neutralize stomach acid

   C) to prevent food materials and stomach acid from leaking into other bodily tissues

   D) to begin the process of chemical digestion

20. Which of the following is the location of fertilization in the female?

   A) uterus

   B) fallopian tube

   C) endometrium

   D) fimbriae

21. The pineal gland is located in which of the following areas in the body?

   A) below the larynx

   B) above the kidney

   C) at the center of the brain hemispheres

   D) at the base of the brain

22. Which of the following processes aids scientists in observing a population sample in order to answer questions about the whole population?

   A) univariate analysis

   B) inferential statistics

   C) descriptive statistics

   D) probability

23. Which of the following biological macromolecules is non-soluble, composed of hydrocarbons, and acts as an important source of energy storage for the body?

   A) carbohydrates

   B) nucleic acids

   C) lipids

   D) proteins

24. Which of the following is specialized tissue in the right atrium that acts as the heart's natural pacemaker by generating the electrical signal for the heartbeat?

   A) sinus venosus

   B) sinoatrial node

   C) atrioventricular node

   D) septa

25. Which of the following is a dense, interconnected mass of nerve cells located outside of the central nervous system?

   A) ganglion

   B) dendrite

   C) cranial nerve

   D) pons

26. Which of the following is the primary cell found in the tract of the small intestine?

   A) surface absorptive cells

   B) surface lining cells

   C) parietal cells

   D) hepatocytes

27. Specialized cells called osteoblasts form new bone tissue through deposition of calcium in which of the following processes?

   A) calcification

   B) osteoporosis

   C) ossification

   D) hematopoiesis

28. Which of the following describes the general function of cytokines in the immune system?

   A) They communicate between cells to instigate an immune response.

   B) They inhibit blood clotting during inflammation responses.

   C) They bind to specific pathogens to increase pathogen mass.

   D) They transport pathogens trapped in mucus to be destroyed in the stomach.

29. Which of the following describes the path through which air moves during inhalation?

   A) mouth/nose > pharynx > larynx > trachea > bronchi > bronchioles > alveoli

   B) bronchioles > alveoli > bronchi > larynx > pharynx > lungs

   C) mouth/nose > bronchi > bronchioles > alveoli > lungs > trachea

   D) alveoli > bronchioles > lungs > bronchi > trachea > larynx > pharynx > mouth/nose

30. Which of the following is not a function of progesterone in the female reproductive system?

   A) expression of secondary sexual characteristics, such as enlarged breasts

   B) stimulation of milk production in the breasts

   C) regulation and preparation of the endometrial lining of the uterus for potential pregnancy

   D) inhibition of contractions of the uterus as the ovum is released

31. Which of the following layers of skin acts as an energy reserve by storing adipocytes and releasing them into circulation when energy is needed?

   A) epidermis

   B) dermis

   C) hypodermis

   D) stratum basale

32. Neurotransmitters send chemical messages across the gap between one neuron and another in which of the following structures?

   A) cell membrane

   B) ganglion

   C) synapse

   D) axon

33. Hund's rule states which of the following?

   A) Chemical bonds are formed only between electrons with similar spin.

   B) The attraction between electrons holds atoms together.

   C) A ground state atom always has a completely filled valence shell.

   D) Electrons fill orbitals singly and with similar spin before pairing.

34. Which of the following is the primary function of the large intestine?

   A) absorbing digested material into the blood

   B) nutrient processing and metabolizing

   C) absorbing water and compacting material into solid waste

   D) bile production and storage

The next three questions are based on the following passage.

A scientist designs an experiment to test the hypothesis that exposure to more sunlight will increase the growth rate of elodea, a type of aquatic plant. The scientist has accumulated data from previous experiments that identify the average growth rate of elodea exposed to natural sunlight in the wild.

In the experiment set up, there are three tanks housing ten elodea each. Tank A is positioned in front of a window to receive natural sunlight similar to what elodea are exposed to; tank B is positioned in front of the same window but has an additional sunlight-replicating lamp affixed to it; and tank C is positioned in a dark corner with no exposure to natural sunlight.

35. When setting up the above experiment, the scientist has the option of using a separate water filter for each of the three tanks or using a single filtration system that attaches all three and affects them simultaneously. Which of the following filter set ups makes a more valid experiment and why?

   A) separate filters for each of the three tanks, because this ensures a higher quality of water for each tank

   B) one filtration system for all three tanks, because this makes filtration a controlled variable

   C) one filtration system for all three tanks, because this reduces the workload for the researcher

   D) separate filters for each of the three tanks, because this adds another variable to be tested and analyzed for inclusion in the experiment's results

36. The above experimental design description is an example of which of the following types of experiments?

   A) field experiment
   B) natural experiment
   C) controlled experiment
   D) observational study

37. Which of the following is the control group in the above experiment?

   A) tank A
   B) tank B
   C) tank C
   D) There is no control group in this experiment.

38. Which of the following is a type of white blood cell that plays a key role in adaptive immunity by seeking out, attacking, and destroying targeted pathogens?

   A) B cells
   B) goblet cells
   C) antibodies
   D) T cells

39. Which of the following are the blood vessels that transport blood to the heart?

   A) arteries
   B) capillaries
   C) venules
   D) veins

40. Which of the following cell organelles are the site of lipid synthesis?

   A) smooth endoplasmic reticulum
   B) ribosome
   C) rough endoplasmic reticulum
   D) Golgi apparatus

41. Which of the following describes a series of measurements that produces exact results on a consistent basis?

A) accurate

B) precise

C) valid

D) significant

42. Chromatids divide into identical chromosomes and migrate to opposite ends of the cell in which of the following phases of mitosis?

A) metaphase

B) anaphase

C) prophase

D) telophase

43. A series of muscle contractions that transports food down the digestive tract in a wave-like fashion describes which of the following?

A) digestion

B) deglutition

C) defecation

D) peristalsis

44. Which of the following is NOT a function of the liver?

A) nutrient processing

B) blood filtration and detoxification

C) cholesterol and lipoprotein production

D) insulin production and blood sugar regulation

45. $2C_6H_{14} + 19O_2 \rightarrow 12CO_2 + 14H_2O$

The reaction above is an example of which of the following?

A) substitution reaction

B) acid-base reaction

C) enzyme reaction

D) combustion reaction

46. Which of the following are regions of the digestive system in which amylase is produced?

A) pancreas and salivary glands

B) gall bladder and salivary glands

C) gall bladder and liver

D) pancreas and liver

47. Which of the following describes a cell's reaction to being placed in a hypertonic solution?

A) The cell will shrink as water is pulled out of the cell to equalize the concentrations inside and outside of the cell.

B) The cell will swell as water is pulled into the cell to equalize the concentrations inside and outside of the cell.

C) The cell will remain the same size since the concentrations inside and outside the cell are equal to begin with.

D) The pH inside the cell will drop in order to equalize the pH inside and outside the cell.

48. Which of the following are the two major zones of the respiratory system?

A) left bronchus and right bronchus

B) nose and mouth

C) larynx and pharynx

D) conducting and respiratory

49. Which of the following is not one of the major tissue layers of the alimentary canal?

A) submucosa

B) muscularis

C) adventitia

D) duodenum

50. Which of the following distinguishes the isotopes of an element?

   A) Isotopes are atoms of the same element that have different ionic charges.

   B) Isotopes are atoms of elements within the same group on the periodic table.

   C) Isotopes are atoms of the same element that have different numbers of neutrons.

   D) Isotopes are atoms of the same element with different electron configurations.

51. Which of the following is the cartilaginous flap that protects the larynx from water or food while still allowing the flow of air?

   A) epiglottis

   B) bronchioles

   C) epithelium

   D) tongue

52. Which of the following describes the function of the fascia in muscle tissue?

   A) to enclose, protect, support, and separate muscle tissue

   B) to connect muscle tissue to bone

   C) to serve as the contractile unit of muscle

   D) to slide past the actin protein cells in muscle to create contraction

53. Which of the following correctly describes a strong acid?

   A) A strong acid completely ionizes in water.

   B) A strong acid donates more than one proton.

   C) A strong acid contains at least one metal atom.

   D) A strong acid will not decompose.

English and Language Usage

Directions: Read the question carefully, and choose the best answer.

1. Which of the following sentences follows the rules of capitalization?

   A) As juveniles, african white-backed vultures are darkly colored, developing their white feathers only as they grow into adulthood.

   B) Ukrainians celebrate a holiday called *Malanka* during which men dress in costumes and masks and play tricks on their neighbors.

   C) Because of its distance from the sun, the planet neptune has seasons that last the equivalent of forty-one earth years.

   D) Edward Jenner, considered the Father of immunology, invented the world's first vaccine.

2. Which of the following would NOT be an acceptable way to revise and combine the underlined portion of the sentences below?

   First and foremost, they receive an annual pension payment. The amount of the pension has been reviewed and changed a number of times, most recently to reflect the salary of a high-level government executive.

   A) annual pension payment, the amount of which

   B) annual pension payment; the amount of the pension

   C) annual pension payment; over the years since 1958, the amount of the pension

   D) annual pension payment, the amount of the pension

3. Which of the following sentences has the correct subject-verb agreement?

   A) The Akhal-Teke horse breed, originally from Turkmenistan, have long enjoyed a reputation for bravery and fortitude.

   B) The employer decided that he could not, due to the high cost of healthcare, afford to offer other benefits to his employees.

   C) Though Puerto Rico is known popularly for its beaches, its landscape also include mountains, which play home to many of the island's rural villages.

   D) Each of the storm chasers decide whether or not to go out when rain makes visibility low.

4. Which of the following is a compound sentence?

   A) Plague, generally not a major public health concern, actually continues to spread among rodent populations today, and it even occasionally makes its way into a human host.

   B) Modern archeology, which seeks answers to humanity's questions about its past, is helped significantly by new technologies.

   C) In the fight against obesity, countries around the world are imposing taxes on sodas and other sugary drinks in an effort to curb unhealthy habits.

   D) Because the assassination of President John F. Kennedy continues to haunt and fascinate Americans, new movies, books, and television series about it are being released every year.

5. Which of the following would most likely be found in an academic research paper on the world's food supply?

A) It's ridiculous that so many people in the world are hungry while others just throw away tons of uneaten food.

B) I've always believed that it's our moral duty as a people to provide food and clean water to those who do not have access to it, which is why I have made research of the food supply my life's work.

C) Advances in agricultural technology over the past five decades have led to a steady increase in the global food supply, and the populations of many countries around the world are benefitting.

D) Poor people should appeal to their governments for help feeding their families.

6. Which of the following is the complete subject in the sentence?

Sandra's principal reason for choosing the job was that it would be full-time and would offer benefits.

A) Sandra's principal reason for choosing the job

B) Sandra's principal reason

C) Sandra's principal

D) Sandra

7. James had already been awake for nineteen hours___ after a twelve-hour work day, when he received the news.

A) .

B) ;

C) ,

D) —

8. Which of the following is a synonym for *prized* as used in the sentence?

Parrots, among the most intelligent birds in the world, have been prized pets for many centuries; in fact, the first recorded instance of parrot training was written in the thirteenth century.

A) unlikely

B) misunderstood

C) rewarded

D) valued

9. Which of the following prefixes would be used to indicate that something is *inside* or *within*?

A) intra–

B) trans–

C) anti–

D) hyper–

10. Which of the following is correctly punctuated?

A) The artist Prince, whose death shocked America in April of 2016; was one of the most successful musical artists of the last century.

B) The artist Prince, whose death shocked America in April of 2016, was one of the most successful musical artists of the last century.

C) The artist Prince—whose death shocked America in April of 2016, was one of the most successful musical artists of the last century.

D) The artist Prince, whose death shocked America in April of 2016: was one of the most successful musical artists of the last century.

11. Which of the following is misspelled in the sentence below?

> Everyday items like potatos, bread, onions, and even saliva are the tools of art conservators, who work to clean and restore works of art.

A) potatos

B) saliva

C) conservators

D) restore

12. Which of the following is an appropriate synonym for *disciplines* as it is used in the sentence?

> The American Academy of Arts and Sciences includes members whose topics of study span many disciplines such as math, science, arts, humanities, public affairs, and business.

A) locations

B) regions

C) punishments

D) fields

13. Which of the following is misspelled in the sentence?

> Today, astrophysicists study the same stars that were observed by the astronemers of the ancient world, though today's techniques and technology are much more advanced.

A) astrophysicists

B) astronemers

C) techniques

D) technology

14. Which of the following nouns is written in the correct plural form?

A) vertebraes

B) gooses

C) octopusses

D) bronchi

15. Which of the following is a complex sentence?

A) When skywriting, a pilot flies a small aircraft in specific, particular formations, creating large letters visible from the ground.

B) The public defense attorney was able to maintain her optimism despite her dearth of courtroom wins, her lack of free time, and her growing list of clients.

C) Because the distance between stars in the galaxy is far greater than the distance between planets, interstellar travel is expected to be an even bigger challenge than interplanetary exploration.

D) Invented in France in the early nineteenth century, the stethoscope underwent a number of reiterations before the emergence of the modern form of the instrument in the 1850s.

16. Which of the following sentences is irrelevant as part of a paragraph composed of these sentences?

A) Traffic around the arena was heavy, so we were worried we'd miss the opening pitch.

B) My brother and I won tickets in a radio station contest to see his favorite team play on opening day.

C) To win the contest, you had to be the 395th caller and know the answer to a trivia question; we waited anxiously by the phone for the contest to begin.

D) My brother has followed the team since childhood, so we knew he'd be able to answer the trivia question correctly.

17.

Table 12.3. Outlines

I. Types of Engines
   A. Heat Engines
      i. Combustion Engines
      ii. Non-Combustion Heat Engines
   B. Electric Engines
   C. Physically Powered Motors
      i. Pneumatic Motors
      ii Hydraulic Motors

Which of the following statements is true regarding the outline?

A) Heat engines are the most common type of engine.

B) Pneumatic and hydraulic motors are both types of electric engines.

C) The three types of engines are heat engines, electric engines, and pneumatic motors.

D) Heat engines can be broken down into combustion and non-combustion engines.

18. In the sentence, the prefix *pre–* indicates that the evaluation will take place at which of the following times?

The patient's preoperative evaluation is scheduled for next Wednesday.

A) before the operation

B) after the operation

C) during the operation

D) at the end of the operation

19. Which of the following root words would be used in a word related to the body?

A) corp

B) auto

C) man

D) bio

20. Which of the following is an appropriate synonym for *traditional* as it is used in the sentence?

Unlike a traditional comic book, a graphic novel is released as one single publication, either in the form of one long story or in the form of an anthology.

A) old-fashioned

B) conventional

C) expensive

D) popular

21. Which of the following words from the sentence is slang?

Her new tennis racket cost her a hundred bucks, but it was worth the steep price tag.

A) cost

B) bucks

C) steep

D) tag

22. Which of the following parts of speech is *widely* as used in the sentence?

Though professional dental care is widely available in the developed world, the prevalence of cavities is much higher there.

A) adjective

B) noun

C) adverb

D) verb

23. Which of the following parts of speech is *remains* as used in the sentence?

Typically, water that has evaporated remains in the sky in cloud form for less than ten days before falling to Earth again as precipitation.

A) noun

B) verb

C) adjective

D) adverb

24. Which of the following punctuation marks is used incorrectly?

Though the term *nomad* is often associated with early populations, nomadic cultures exist today, especially in the mountain's of Europe and Asia.

A) the comma after *populations*

B) the comma after *today*

C) the apostrophe in *mountain's*

D) the period after *Asia*

25. Which of the following punctuation marks is used incorrectly?

On Parents' Day, a public holiday in the Democratic Republic of Congo, families celebrate parents' both living and deceased.

A) the apostrophe in *Parents' Day*

B) the comma following *Day*

C) the comma following *Congo*

D) the apostrophe in *parents'*

26. Which is the best way to revise and combine the underlined portion of the sentences?

Unfortunately, the belief that changelings could be convinced to leave was not just <u>an innocuous superstition. On some occasions,</u> harm came to the individual who was thought to be a changeling.

A) an innocuous superstition, on some occasions,

B) an innocuous superstition, but on some occasions,

C) an innocuous superstition; however, on some occasions,

D) an innocuous superstition: on some occasions,

27. Which of the following phrases follows the rules of capitalization?

A) President Carter and his advisors

B) Robert Jones, the senior Senator from California

C) my Aunt and Uncle who live out west

D) the party on New Year's eve

28. Which of the following sentences has correct pronoun-antecedent agreement?

A) The storm, which included three days of rain, was very strong, and they left half the city flooded.

B) Each of the cars needs to be examined for damage by a mechanic; he may need repairs.

C) The number of people who had to evacuate hasn't been confirmed, but it is small.

D) Many people were able to take advantage of shelters, where he or she was kept safe from the storm.

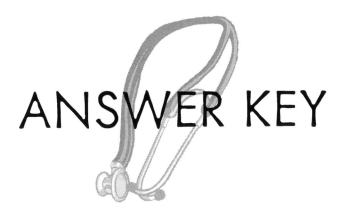

ANSWER KEY

Mathematics

1. **C)**

   First calculate 20% of the list price:

   $0.20 \times \$26,580 = \$5,316$

   Next calculate the savings over the first 3 months of payments:

   3 months × \$250/month = \$750

   Find the total savings:

   $\$5,316 + \$750 = \$6,066$

2. **C)**

   First find the total cost before tax:

   5 shirts × \$3/shirt + 4 pants × \$6/pants + 2 items mended × \$5/item mended = \$49

   Now multiply this amount by 1.08 to account for the added 8% sales tax:

   $\$49 \times 1.08 = \$52.92$

3. **A)**

   Let s be the number of sandwiches sold. Each sandwich earns \$4, so selling s sandwiches at \$4 each results in revenue of \$4s. Similarly, d drinks at \$2 each gives \$2d of income and cookies bring in \$1c. Summing these values gives a total of revenue = $4s + 2d + 1c$. The correct answer is A).

4. **C)**

   The y-intercept will have an x value of 0. This eliminates choices A), B) and D). Plug $x = 0$ into the equation and solve for y to find the y-intercept:

   $7y - 42(0) + 7 = 0$, so $7y = -7$ and therefore $y = -1$. The correct answer is $(0, -1)$, which is answer C).

5. **C)**

   First complete the operations in parentheses: $4 - \frac{1}{2^2} + 24 \div (8 + 12) = 4 - \frac{1}{2^2} + 24 \div (20)$

   Next simplify the exponents: $4 - \frac{1}{2^2} + 24 \div (20) = 4 - \frac{1}{4} + 24 \div (20)$

   Then complete multiplication and division operations: $4 - \frac{1}{4} + 24 \div (20) = 4 - 0.25 + 1.2$

   Finally complete addition and subtraction operations:

   $4 - 0.25 + 1.2 = 4.95$

6. **A)**

   The area of a rectangle is *length × width*, so $A = L(3L)$. The area was given, so

   $1452 = 3L^2$

   Solving for L: $484 = L^2$ and $L = \pm 22$.

   Since length must be positive, $L = 22$ feet.

7. **A)**

Calculate the decline:

40% decline in 70% of the business = $0.40 \times 0.70 = 0.28 = 28\%$ decline

Calculate the growth:

60% growth in 25% of the business = $0.60 \times 0.25 = 0.15 = 15\%$ growth

Find the net change:

28% decline + 15% growth = $-0.28 + 0.15$ = $-0.13 = 13\%$ decline

8. **D)**

The first step is to multiply (resulting in 17.92); then divide the result by 0.4 (making 44.80 the solution).

9. **B)**

First convert the dimensions to meters:

$15 \text{ ft.} \times \dfrac{1 \text{ m}}{3.28 \text{ ft.}} = 4.57 \text{ m}$

$9 \text{ ft.} \times \dfrac{1 \text{ m}}{3.28 \text{ ft.}} = 2.74 \text{ m}$

$12.5 \text{ ft.} \times \dfrac{1 \text{ m}}{3.28 \text{ ft.}} = 3.81 \text{ m}$

Next find the total area in square meters:

total area = $2(4.57 \text{ m} \times 2.74 \text{ m}) + 2(3.81 \text{ m} \times 2.74 \text{ m}) = 45.9 \text{ m}^2$

Finally convert the area to gallons of paint:

$45.9 \text{ m}^2 \times \dfrac{1 \text{ gallon}}{32 \text{ m}^2} = 1.43 \text{ gallons}$

10. **D)**

First convert mixed fractions to improper fractions:

$5\frac{2}{3} \times 1\frac{7}{8} \div \frac{1}{3} = \frac{17}{3} \times \frac{15}{8} \div \frac{1}{3}$

Next flip the divisor fraction and multiply:

$\frac{17}{3} \times \frac{15}{8} \div \frac{1}{3} = \frac{17}{3} \times \frac{15}{8} \times \frac{3}{1} =$

$\frac{17 \times 15 \times 3}{3 \times 8 \times 1} = \frac{765}{24}$

Now divide the numerator by the denominator to convert back to a mixed fraction:

$\frac{765}{24} = 31\frac{21}{24}$

Finally find the greatest common factor to reduce the fraction:

$31\frac{21}{24} = 31\frac{21 \div 3}{24 \div 3} = 31\frac{7}{8}$

11. **D)**

A $\frac{3}{20}$ increase means the new wage is $w + w\left(\frac{3}{20}\right)$, or $w\left(1 + \frac{3}{20}\right)$.

Convert the fraction to decimal form:

$\frac{3}{20} = \frac{3}{20}\left(\frac{5}{5}\right) = \frac{15}{100} = 0.15$

The new wage is:

$w(1 + 0.15) = 1.15w$

12. **C)**

In algebraic terms, the ratio can be expressed with the following equation:

$9x + 2x + 1x = 36$

Here, x represents some common factor by which each number of employees was divided to reduce the ratio. Solve for x, then find $2x$ to solve for the number of hosts:

$9x + 2x + 1x = 36$

$12x = 36$

$x = 3$

$2x = 2 \times 3 = 6$

13. **C)**

$(1 - x)$ = proportion of men who do not play an instrument

$(1 - x) = \dfrac{\text{number of men who do not play an instrument}}{z}$

$(1 - x)z$ = number of men who do not play an instrument

14. **D)**

Adding 20% is equivalent to paying 120% of the bill:

$\$48.30 \times \frac{120}{100} = \$57.96$

15. **C)**

Convert the fractions to decimals:

$\frac{6}{9} \approx 0.67$

$\frac{1}{7} \approx 0.14$

Now order the numbers from smallest to largest:

$0.125 < 0.14 < 0.60 < 0.67$

16. **D)**

Because the last decimal digit is in the hundredths place, the decimal part of the number is written as a fraction over 100. The fraction of $\frac{28}{100}$ reduces to $\frac{7}{25}$.

17. **B)**

Start by multiplying both sides by 7:

$7(x \div 7) = 7(x - 36)$

$x = 7x - 252$

Now subtract $7x$ from both sides:

$x - 7x = 7x - 252 - 7x$

$-6x = -252$

Finally divide both sides by −6:

$\dfrac{-6x}{-6} = \dfrac{-252}{-6}$

$x = 42$

18. **B)**

A proportion is written using two ratios relating amount earned to months, with x representing the unknown amount:

$\dfrac{15{,}036}{7} = \dfrac{x}{2}$.

The proportion is solved by cross-multiplying and dividing: $7x = 30{,}072$, $x = 4{,}296$. The solution is $4,296.

19. **B)**

The cost c of gas has units dollars per mile. Construct an expression that yields these units:

$$p/m = \frac{\left(\frac{\$}{\text{gal.}}\right)}{\left(\frac{\text{mi.}}{\text{gal.}}\right)} = \frac{(\$)\cancel{(\text{gal.})}}{(\text{mi.})\cancel{(\text{gal.})}} = \frac{\$}{\text{mi.}}$$

20. **C)**

Use the area to find the length of one side of the square:

$A = l \times w = l^2$

$5{,}625 \text{ ft.}^2 = l^2$

$l = \sqrt{5{,}625 \text{ ft.}^2} = 75 \text{ ft.}$

Now multiply the side length by 4 to find the perimeter:

$P = 4l$

$P = 4(75 \text{ ft.}) = 300 \text{ ft.}$

21. **B)**

Find the area of all of the sides of the shed. Two walls measure 5 feet by 7 feet; the other two walls measure 4 feet by 7 feet:

$A = 2l_1w_1 + 2l_2w_2$

$A = 2(5 \text{ ft.})(7 \text{ ft.}) + 2(4 \text{ ft.})(7 \text{ ft.})$

$A = 70 \text{ ft.}^2 + 56 \text{ ft.}^2 = 126 \text{ ft.}^2$

22. **A)**

The formula for the circumference of a circle is:

$C = 2\pi r$

Because $d = 2r$, this formula can be rewritten:

$C = \pi d$

$49 \text{ ft.} = \pi d$

$d = \dfrac{49 \text{ ft.}}{\pi} = 15.6 \text{ ft.}$

23. **D)**

To find the median, first order the data points from smallest to largest:

17, 25, 38, 41, 42, 45, 46, 50

There is an even number of data points. Locate the middle two points and take the average:

~~17, 25, 38,~~ 41, 42, ~~45, 46, 50~~

$(41 + 42) \div 2 = 41.5$

24. **C)**

Find Sam's income for each month:

January: $900

February: $1100

March: $500

April: $200

May: $400

Now find the average by adding those values and dividing by 5. Then round to the nearest 100:

$\dfrac{900 + 1100 + 500 + 200 + 400}{5} = 620 \approx 600$

25. **B)**

Since there are 16 ounces in a pound, 8 ounces = 0.5 pounds. The conversion factor of kilograms to pounds is therefore multiplied by 8.5 pounds. The calculation is:

$8.5 \text{ lb.}\left(\dfrac{1 \text{ kg}}{2.2 \text{ lb.}}\right) = \dfrac{8.5}{2.2} = 3.9 \text{ kg.}$

Notice that the 1 is on top in this conversion factor so that pounds cancel. The unit that the quantity is being converted to must always be in the numerator.

26. **D)**

To add or subtract numbers in scientific notation, the exponents of the base of 10 must be the same. The first number can be rewritten as $4.71 \times 10 \times 10^2 =$ 47.1×10^2. The values in front of 10^2 are subtracted, and the power of 10 stays the same, with a result of 44.12×10^2. The solution is then rewritten in proper scientific notation as 4.412×10^3.

27. **B)**

The answer choices are −6, 0, −11, and −30 for A), B), C), and D), respectively. Answer choice B), 0, is the only response that is not negative.

28. **D)**

The algebraic expression can be simplified using PEMDAS.

$10^2 - 7(3 - 4) - 25 \rightarrow$

$10^2 - 7(-1) - 25 \rightarrow$

$100 + 7 - 25 \rightarrow$

$107 - 25 \rightarrow$

82

29. **B)**

The algebraic expression can be simplified using PEMDAS.

$\dfrac{5^2(3) + 3(-2)^2}{4 + 3^2 - 2(5 - 8)} = \dfrac{5^2(3) + 3(-2)^2}{4 + 3^2 - 2(-3)} \rightarrow$

$\dfrac{25(3) + 3(4)}{4 + 9 - 2(-3)} = \dfrac{75 + 12}{13 + 6} = \dfrac{87}{19}$

30. **C)**

First convert everything to kilograms:

$800 \text{ g} \times \dfrac{1 \text{ kg}}{1000 \text{ g}} = 0.8 \text{ kg}$

$300 \text{ g} \times \dfrac{1 \text{ kg}}{1000 \text{ g}} = 0.3 \text{ kg}$

Next find the total weight:

$1.2 \text{ kg} + 0.8 \text{ kg} + 0.3 \text{ kg} = 2.3 \text{ kg}$

Now find the total cost by multiplying by $4/kg:

$2.3 \text{ kg} \times \dfrac{\$4}{1 \text{ kg}} = \$9.20$

31. **B)**

Each fraction is changed to an improper fraction: $\left(\dfrac{3}{2}\right)\left(\dfrac{8}{3}\right) \div \dfrac{5}{4}$.

Using PEMDAS and working left to right:

$\left(\dfrac{3}{2}\right)\left(\dfrac{8}{3}\right) \div \dfrac{5}{4} = \dfrac{24}{6} \div \dfrac{5}{4} = \dfrac{4}{1} \div \dfrac{5}{4}$.

To divide the fractions, the second fraction is flipped and then multiplied by the first fraction, giving $\left(\dfrac{4}{1}\right)\left(\dfrac{4}{5}\right) = \dfrac{16}{5}$.

This simplifies to $3\dfrac{1}{5}$.

32. **D)**

First, simplify the exponents:

$2^{-1} = \dfrac{1}{2^1} = \dfrac{1}{2}$

$(-1)^3 = -1$

Now, order the quantities from most negative to most positive:

$-\dfrac{4}{3}, -1, \dfrac{2}{5}, \dfrac{1}{2}$

33. **C)**

The digit in the tenths place is 7 and is rounded up to 8 because the digit in the hundredths place is 8, which is greater than or equal to 5. So the number is rounded up to 2.8.

34. **C)**

A proportion is solved by cross-multiplying:

$5(4x - 5) = \dfrac{3}{2}(2x - 6)$

Then, the linear equation is solved for x:

$20x - 25 = 3x - 9;\ 17x = 16;\ x = \dfrac{16}{17}$.

35. **D)**

Start by adding 6 to both sides:

$8x - 6 + 6 = 3x + 24 + 6$

$8x = 3x + 30$

Next subtract $3x$ from both sides:

$8x - 3x = 3x + 30 - 3x$

$5x = 30$

Finally divide both sides by 5 to solve for x:

$5x \div 5 = 30 \div 5$

$x = 6$

36. **D)**

The solution can be written as a fraction by dividing the number of correct questions by the total number of questions:

$\dfrac{42}{48} = 0.875$

Then, the result is multiplied by 100 for a grade of 87.5%.

Reading

1. **B) is correct.** The purpose of the passage is to explain what an idealist believes in. The author does not offer any opinions or try to persuade readers about the importance of certain values.

2. **A) is correct.** The systolic blood pressure is the higher number marked as "Sys" on the monitor.

3. **D) is correct.** The loyal dog is presented in contrast with humans, who are not always trustworthy or faithful.

4. **A) is correct.** The author is describing the constancy of dogs as friends. He concludes by stating, "When all other friends desert, he [a dog] remains."

5. **C) is correct.** The passage emphasizes that people can be treacherous, but a dog will be a constant friend. The passage does not suggest that relationships with other people are pointless or useless.

6. **D) is correct.** The author is trying to persuade his audience that dogs are loyal friends.

7. **B) is correct.** The first step in the *After Planting* section is to water the plants immediately.

8. **A) is correct.** In the *Before Planting* section, the directions say to mix in fertilizer or compost after the soil has been loosened.

9. **C) is correct.** The author and Alan have a friendly relationship, as evidenced by the author's casual tone and his offer to bring Alan a gift from his vacation.

10. **C) is correct.** The author is writing to tell Alan that he will be out of the office. The details about his trip and the meeting support this idea.

11. **B) is correct.** The Scout Camp is due north of the Fire Circle.

12. **A) is correct.** The Old Oak Tree lies on the trail between the Fishing Pond and the Fire Circle.

13. **D) is correct.** The author wants to bring customers into Carl's Car Depot, doing so by highlighting the low prices and range of cars available.

14. **B) is correct.** The word *sell* best describes the author's implication that the cars are priced to be sold quickly.

15. **A) is correct.** The passage does not mention warranties.

16. **C) is correct.** The word *said* is italicized to provide emphasis and contrast with the word actions.

17. **A) is correct.** Choice A describes the order of Julia's actions that matches chronological order of the passage.

18. **B) is correct.** The passage describes how Julia had an exhausting morning, and it can be assumed that when "she'd had enough" she decided to go home.

19. **C) is correct.** Whether or not it was irresponsible for Julia to leave work is a matter of opinion. Some readers may agree, and others may disagree. The other statements are facts that can be proven from the passage.

20. **B) is correct.** The phrase "set a course for home" is an idiom that means to head in a certain direction, so Julia is planning to go home.

21. **D) is correct.** The passage emphasizes that Julia is tired, so she's most likely to drive home and go to sleep.

22. **D) is correct.** In the passage, Thomas Jefferson is defined as an anti-Federalist, in contrast with Federalists who believe in a strong federal government.

23. **B) is correct.** *Tropical Frogs* belongs under the heading *Frogs* with the other types of frogs. The blank spot should not include a specific type of frog or refer to amphibians other than frogs.

24. **A) is correct.** Only Choice A is a source produced by someone who does not have first-hand experience of World War I.

25. **A) is correct.** Victoria's win implies that she played in a competitive event.

26. **D) is correct.** Quarter Price Books has the lowest price: $(3.99 \times 25) + (2.99 \times 50) = 249.25$

27. **B) is correct.** The Book Barn would offer the lowest price: $98 for twenty-five books.

28. **A) is correct.** A company that profits from private tutoring might introduce bias into a study on the effects of private tutoring in schools.

29. **C) is correct.** The author cites data from a study to support his or her argument.

30. **C) is correct.** Choice C shows the correct order of the blocks after following the directions.

31. **D) is correct.** Choice D correctly lists the houses the author visited as listed chronologically in the passage.

32. **B) is correct.** The author says that the house on Pine Street "had enough space inside but didn't have a big enough yard for our three dogs."

33. **B) is correct.** A local paper is the source most likely to provide an unbiased assessment of the candidates in a state election.

34. **D) is correct.** The passage concludes with the statement "our Human Resources team will be taking longer than previously stated to review candidates and schedule interviews"

and a time window in which Mr. Morgan can expect to receive feedback.

35. **A) is correct.** The author of the passage states that the team will be taking "longer than previously stated," implying that she had previously told Mr. Morgan that the process would take less than two weeks.

36. **C) is correct.** The passage states that babies' senses are much like those of their adult counterparts with the exception of their vision, which develops later.

37. **B) is correct.** The passage states that "infants rely primarily on hearing."

38. **A) is correct.** The passage explains how a baby's senses develop and allow it to interact with the world.

39. **C) is correct.** Ginger appears on the list for fall.

40. **D) is correct.** The word *given* best describes the idea that the gifts have been handed out.

41. **B) is correct.** Only Choice B includes the fact that both Epimetheus and Prometheus were assigned to create living things; it then clarifies that Epimetheus gave positive traits to animals, while Prometheus gave fire to humans. This choice includes all the important parts of the passage without adding other emotions or details.

42. **B) is correct.** *Lamb* fits best with the pattern of subheadings naming specific types of meat.

43. **A) is correct.** Page 55 is included in the section on Italian painters.

44. **C) is correct.** Page 153 is the beginning of the section on High Renaissance architecture, which includes the year 1518.

45. **D) is correct.** The passage states that restaurateurs must be "exact and

ruthless with their budget and pricing."
The success of The Hot Dog implies that
its owners have done that.

46. **D) is correct.** *Evidence* best describes
the idea that The Hot Dog's longevity is
proof of its owners' skills.

47. **B) is correct.** In February the service
earned $1100, and in April it earned
$200. The difference between the two
months is $900.

48. **B) is correct.** The author uses several
markers of casual writing, including the
first person, exclamation marks, and
informal language.

49. **C) is correct.** The diagram indicates
that products are formed when the
substrate is broken apart.

50. **C) is correct.** The transition word
finally indicates that it is the end of a
sequence.

51. **A) is correct.** The index shows that the
Battle of the Scheldt appears on page
110.

Science

1. **B) is correct.** Oxygen intake and carbon dioxide disposal are the primary functions of the respiratory system.

2. **B) is correct.** Making observations is the first step of the scientific method; observations enable the researcher to form a question and begin the research process.

3. **D) is correct.** The mechanism of natural selection is rooted in the idea that there is variation in inherited traits among a population of organisms, and that there is differential reproduction as a result.

4. **A) is correct.** Gonadotrophs produce both FSH and LH, which play a key role in ovulation, lactation, sperm development, and testosterone production.

5. **B) is correct.** Ovarian follicles each contain a sac with an immature egg, or oocyte. During the female reproductive cycle, several oocytes will mature into a mature ovum. Eventually, one ovum is released per cycle during ovulation.

6. **B) is correct.** The tongue is a muscle that plays a primary role in digestion and, in conjunction with teeth, prepares food for swallowing.

7. **A) is correct.** The left atrium receives oxygenated blood, then moves it downward into the left ventricle.

8. **C) is correct.** The parietal lobe is considered the primary sensory processing and integrating center of the brain.

9. **C) is correct.** The humoral immune response is characterized by the mediation and production of antibodies. In this adaptive response, B lymphocytes recognize and attach pathogens together to prevent dispersal.

10. **A) is correct.** Data is considered reliable if similar results are found after repeated experiments following consistent conditions; however, if data does not accurately measure the variable it is intended to measure, it is not considered valid.

11. **C) is correct.** Mendel's law of independent assortment, his second law of heredity, expands on the law of segregation by stipulating that alleles which separate in the gamete stage do so independently of other genes.

12. **B) is correct.** Proceeding top to bottom on the periodic table, atoms gain more and more layers of electrons in their orbitals, increasing radius. Proceeding right to left on the periodic table, atoms have fewer valence electrons and the attraction between nucleus and electrons decreases. Both of these effects cause a trend of increasing radius down and to the left on the periodic table.

13. **C) is correct.** Enamel is a tissue found in teeth, but not skeletal bones.

14. **B) is correct.** Semilunar valves are present in the pulmonary trunk and the aortic trunk; they allow blood to enter the vessels and prevent its return back to the heart.

15. **D) is correct.** Neuromuscular junctions are the location in which the nervous system communicates with the muscular system to create muscle contraction and movement.

16. **A) is correct.** Calcium is the most abundant mineral found in bones, as well as the entire body.

17. **B) is correct.** The medulla oblongata, along with the pons, is a portion of the brain stem that regulates critical body functions.

18. **C) is correct.** The skin, which provides a seamless layer of cells around the entire body, is the primary physical barrier that prevents pathogens from entering the body.

19. **A) is correct.** The pyloric sphincter acts as a valve at the connection of the stomach and small intestine.

20. **B) is correct.** A released ovum stays in the fallopian tube for approximately 24 hours. If sperm have not migrated up the tubes to fertilize the egg, then it moves through the uterus; if fertilization does occur, it stays in the tube for several more days as it moves to the uterus for implantation.

21. **C) is correct.** The pineal gland is located in the epithalamus and is a gland involved in the production of melatonin.

22. **B) is correct.** Inferential statistics are used to analyze and apply data beyond the immediate data from an observation or experiment.

23. **C) is correct.** Lipids, which include but are not limited to fats, are an efficient source of energy storage due to their ability to store nearly twice as much energy as carbohydrates and proteins.

24. **B) is correct.** The sinoatrial (SA) node is an area of specialized muscle tissue in the right atrium that generates an electrical signal which spreads from cell to cell to generate the heartbeat.

25. **A) is correct.** Ganglions are dense clusters of nerve cells responsible for processing sensory information and coordinating motor activity.

26. **A) is correct.** Surface absorptive cells (SAC) line the intestinal microvilli to absorb food material as it passes through the intestine.

27. **C) is correct.** Ossification is the general term referring to the formation or conversion of bone by osteoblasts.

28. **A) is correct.** Cytokines are small proteins released by cells and have a great impact on cell communication and behavior. There are many kinds of cytokines with a great variety of functions; in the immune system, some cytokines play a critical role in immune response activation by triggering inflammation, fever, and other responses.

29. **A) is correct.** This is the path air follows through the respiratory system during gas exchange.

30. **A) is correct.** Expression of secondary sexual characteristics is regulated by estrogen.

31. **C) is correct.** The hypodermis is the thickest layer of skin and is the site of much of the stored fat in the human body.

32. **C) is correct.** Synapses are connections between two neurons. Nerve signals trigger the release of neurotransmitters, which carry the nerve impulse across the synaptic cleft, or gap, between cells, to be received by the receptor site of the next cell.

33. **D) is correct.** Hund's rule states that electrons fill orbitals in a specific order, and they fill orbitals singly with similar spin before pairing.

34. **C) is correct.** The large intestine, or colon, is an s-shaped organ that dehydrates food material as it travels through the organ and is eliminated at the rectum.

35. **B) is correct.** Using one filtration system for all three tanks keeps the water quality across all three tanks constant and eliminates experimental bias for this variable.

36. **C) is correct.** A controlled experiment requires researchers to compare an experimental group with a control group while controlling all variables

except for the independent variable, which the researcher manipulates to test the hypothesis.

37. **A) is correct.** Tank A is the control group because the sunlight variable is unchanged from the sunlight the elodea are exposed to in their natural environment.

38. **D) is correct.** T cells are a type of white blood cell that originates in the thymus. There are four different varieties of mature T cells, each of which serves a different function in the immune system.

39. **D) is correct.** Veins are blood vessels that move blood to the heart using a series of valves.

40. **A) is correct.** The smooth endoplasmic reticulum is a series of membranes attached to the cell nucleus and plays an important role in the production and storage of lipids. It is called smooth because it lacks ribosomes on the membrane surface.

41. **B) is correct.** Precision describes measurements that are consistently close to one another and the average measurement.

42. **B) is correct.** The sister chromatids of each chromosome are pulled apart by the spindle and pulled to opposite centrosomes during anaphase, elongating the cell in the process.

43. **D) is correct.** Peristalsis begins in the esophagus, where the bolus of food material is swallowed, and continues to transport food to the stomach, the small intestine, and the large intestine.

44. **D) is correct.** Insulin production and blood sugar regulation are performed by the pancreas.

45. **D) is correct.** Combustion is defined as a reaction with O_2 in order to produce CO_2 and H_2O.

46. **A) is correct.** Both the pancreas and salivary glands produce amylase, which is an enzyme that helps digest carbohydrates.

47. **A) is correct.** A hypertonic solution has a higher concentration than the interior of the cell, and water will rush out of the cell to equalize the concentrations, causing the cell to shrink.

48. **D) is correct.** The conducting zone consists of the upper respiratory tract from the nose and mouth through the trachea; it filters and conducts air into the lungs. The respiratory zone consists of the lower respiratory tract from the bronchioles to the alveoli and serves as a site of gas exchange.

49. **D) is correct.** The duodenum is a region of the small intestine that neutralizes materials entering from the stomach.

50. **C) is correct.** Isotopes are atoms that differ in their number of neutrons but are otherwise identical.

51. **A) is correct.** The epiglottis is the protective flap at the entrance of the larynx.

52. **A) is correct.** Fascia is connective tissue that encloses individual muscle fibers.

53. **A) is correct.** Strong acids break apart into their constituent ions immediately when placed in water.

English and Language Usage

1. **B) is correct.** Both *Ukrainians* and *Malanka* must be capitalized; both are proper nouns, and *Ukrainians* begins a sentence.

2. **D) is correct.** This choice creates a comma splice.

3. **B) is correct.** The verb is the singular *afford*, and its subject is the singular *employer*.

4. **A) is correct.** Here, two independent clauses are connected by a comma plus the coordinating conjunction *and*.

5. **C) is correct.** This choice uses formal language, the third-person perspective, and non-judgmental language.

6. **A) is correct.** The complete subject includes the main noun (*reason*) and all its accompanying modifying phrases.

7. **C) is correct.** The inessential phrase *after a twelve-hour work day* is being set apart from the rest of the sentence by commas.

8. **D) is correct.** If these intelligent birds have been kept as pets for so long and if people have taken the time to train them, it is most likely that parrots are *valued* animals.

9. **A) is correct.** The prefix *intra–* means *inside* or *within*.

10. **B) is correct.** The inessential appositive phrase *whose death shocked America in April of 2016* is correctly set apart from the rest of the sentence by commas. Choices A and D create sentence fragments, and Choice C incorrectly pairs an em dash with a comma.

11. **A) is correct.** *Potatos* should be spelled *potatoes*.

12. **D) is correct.** *Fields* best describes the idea that members study many different areas of knowledge; furthermore, the word *field* may refer to something intangible. There are many topics of study in many *fields*, or disciplines.

13. **B) is correct.** *Astronemers* should be spelled *astronomers*.

14. **D) is correct.** The noun *bronchus* is made plural by changing the *–us* to *–i*.

15. **C) is correct.** This sentence includes an independent clause (*interstellar travel is expected to be an even bigger challenge than interplanetary exploration*) and a dependent clause (*Because the distance between stars in the galaxy is far greater than the distance between planets*).

16. **A) is correct.** This sentence does not relate to the flow of information provided by the other three, which tell the story of the siblings' experience with the radio contest. It only discusses the siblings' experience attending the game itself.

17. **D) is correct.** The two subheadings under "Heat Engines" are "Combustion Engines" and "Non-Combustion Engines."

18. **A) is correct.** The prefix *pre–* means *before*.

19. **A) is correct.** The root word *corp* means *body*.

20. **B) is correct.** *Conventional* best describes the idea that comic books have an established narrative framework, a main point in the sentence.

21. **B) is correct.** *Bucks* is a slang term for *dollars*.

22. **C) is correct.** *Widely* is an adverb modifying the adjective *available*.

23. **B) is correct.** *Remains* is a verb in the sentence.

24. **C) is correct.** *Mountain's* is not possessive in this sentence, so it does not require an apostrophe.

25. **D) is correct.** The second *parents* is plural, not possessive, so it does not require an apostrophe.

26. **D) is correct.** The colon correctly signifies that the second clause builds on the first.

27. **A) is correct.** *President* is a title and should be capitalized when it precedes a name.

28. **C) is correct.** *Number* is singular, so it agrees with the singular pronoun *it*.

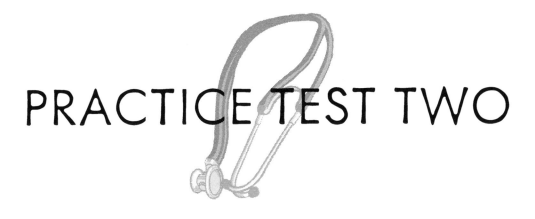

thirteen

PRACTICE TEST TWO

Mathematics

Directions: Read the problem carefully, and choose the best answer.

1. $4x \div (x - 1)$

   Which of the following is the value of the expression above when $x = 5$?

   A) 0

   B) 1

   C) 4

   D) 5

2. Which of the following is the slope of the graph below?

   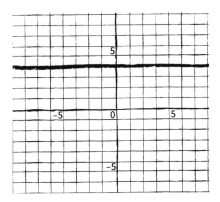

   A) ∞

   B) non-existent

   C) 0

   D) 1

3. Alex, David, and Rachel go out to dinner. Alex and David decide to split an appetizer that costs $8.50, and Rachel gets her own appetizer that costs $6.50. Rachel orders lemonade that costs $3, while Alex and David drink the free water. They all order entrées that cost the same price. They split up the bill according to what each person ordered. Which of the following states how much less Alex and David will pay than Rachel?

   A) $1.00

   B) $5.00

   C) $5.25

   D) $7.25

4. There are 450 students in the tenth grade. Of these, 46% are boys. If 21% of the girls have already turned 16, which of the following is the number of girls in the tenth grade who are 16?

   A) 43

   B) 51

   C) 54

   D) 94

5. A faucet is leaking 1 drop every 4 seconds. If 1 gallon is equal to 15,140 drops, which of the following lengths of time will it take for this faucet to leak 1 gallon of water?

   A) 1 hour, 3 minutes, 5 seconds

   B) 4 hours, 12 minutes, 20 seconds

   C) 16 hours, 49 minutes, 20 seconds

   D) 18 hours, 24 minutes, 5 seconds

6. $(3+5)^2 + 24 \div 16 - 5 \div 2$

   Simplify the expression. Which of the following is correct?

   A) 0.25

   B) 30.25

   C) 33

   D) 63

7. Ashley has been training for a 10-kilometer race. Her average training pace is 8 minutes and 15 seconds per mile. If she maintains this pace during the race, which of the following will be her finishing time? (1 mile = 5280 feet; 1 foot = 0.3048 meters)

   A) 51:23

   B) 50:53

   C) 51:14

   D) 82:30

8. $\frac{8}{15} \div \frac{1}{6}$

   Simplify the expression. Which of the following is correct?

   A) $3\frac{1}{15}$

   B) $\frac{15}{48}$

   C) $\frac{4}{45}$

   D) $3\frac{1}{5}$

9. A marinade recipe calls for 2 tablespoons of lemon juice for $\frac{1}{4}$ cup of olive oil. Which of the following is the amount of lemon juice that should be used with $\frac{2}{3}$ cup olive oil?

   A) $5\frac{1}{3}$ tbsp.

   B) $\frac{3}{4}$ tbsp.

   C) 4 tbsp.

   D) $2\frac{1}{3}$ tbsp.

10. If x represents the proportion of ninth graders in a particular school who are female, and y represents the proportion of students in the school who are ninth graders, which of the following is the expression for the proportion of students in the school who are female ninth graders?

   A) $x + y$

   B) $\frac{x}{y}$

   C) xy

   D) $\frac{y}{x}$

11. Toledo has been working full time but would like to cut back to part time. He normally works from 9:00 a.m. to 5:00 p.m. Monday through Friday. Now he leaves at 1:00 p.m. on Tuesdays and Thursdays. Which of the following is the percentage by which he decreased his weekly work hours?

   A) 20%

   B) 25%

   C) 30%

   D) 80%

12. Which of the following lists is in order from least to greatest?

   A) $\frac{1}{24} < \frac{3}{32} < \frac{5}{48} < \frac{2}{16} < \frac{3}{16}$

   B) $\frac{1}{24} < \frac{5}{48} < \frac{3}{32} < \frac{2}{16} < \frac{3}{16}$

   C) $\frac{1}{24} < \frac{3}{32} < \frac{2}{16} < \frac{3}{16} < \frac{5}{48}$

   D) $\frac{1}{24} < \frac{2}{16} < \frac{3}{32} < \frac{3}{16} < \frac{5}{48}$

13. $3a + 4 = 2a$

Solve the equation. Which of the following is correct?

A) $a = -4$

B) $a = 4$

C) $a = \frac{-4}{5}$

D) $a = \frac{4}{5}$

14. Caroline reads 40 pages in 45 minutes. Which of the following is the approximate number minutes it will take her to read 265 pages?

A) 202 minutes

B) 236 minutes

C) 265 minutes

D) 298 minutes

15. Jane earns $15 per hour babysitting. If she starts out with $275 in her bank account, which of the following equations represents the amount of hours she will need to spend babysitting in order for her account to reach $400?

A) $275 = 400 + 15h$

B) $400 = 15h$

C) $400 = \frac{15}{h} + 275$

D) $400 = 275 + 15h$

16. Which of the following is the total surface area of a box that is 12 inches long, 18 inches wide, and 6 inches high?

A) 144 sq. in.

B) 396 sq. in.

C) 792 sq. in.

D) 1,296 cu. in.

17. Which of the following has the greatest numeric value?

A) $-4(3)(-2)$

B) $-16 - 17 + 31$

C) $18 - 15 + 27$

D) $-20 + 10 + 10$

18. A pizza has a diameter of 10 inches. If a slice with a central angle of 40 degrees is cut from the pizza, which of the following will be the surface area of the pizza slice?

A) 9.2. sq. in.

B) 8.7 sq. in.

C) 3.5 sq. in.

D) 17.4 sq. in.

19. Meg rolled a 6-sided die 4 times, and her first 3 rolls were 1, 3, and 5. If the average of the 4 rolls is 2.5, which of the following was the value of the 4th roll?

A) 1

B) 2

C) 3

D) 5

20. The data set below shows the number of instruments played by students in the seventh and tenth grades. Which of the following is the difference in the average number of instruments played by seventh- and tenth-graders?

Table 13.1. Instruments Played

STUDENT	GRADE	NUMBER OF INSTRUMENTS
Alison	7	2
Dana	10	0
Jerry	7	1
Sam	7	1
Luke	10	1
Philip	7	2
Briana	10	1
Laura	10	0
Angie	7	2

A) 0.5

B) 1

C) 1.1

D) 2.1

21. The pie chart below shows a high school graduating class' enrollment in 4 types of universities: small private, large private, small public, and large public. Of the students who enrolled in a public university, which of the following is the percentage enrolled in a small public university?

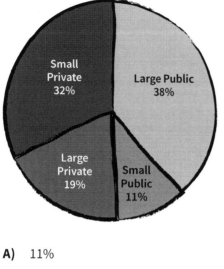

A) 11%

B) 22%

C) 27%

D) 29%

22. If there are 3.28 feet in 1 meter, which of the following is equivalent to 55 meters? (Round to the nearest tenth.)

A) 16.8 feet

B) 21.7 feet

C) 139.7 feet

D) 180.4 feet

23. $-(3)^2 + (5 - 7)^2 - 3(4 - 8)$

Simplify the expression. Which of the following is correct?

A) −17

B) −1

C) 7

D) 25

24. $(3^2 \div 1^3) - (4 - 8^2) + 2^4$

Simplify the expression. Which of the following is correct?

A) −35

B) −4

C) 28

D) 85

25. 17.38 − 19.26 + 14.2

Simplify the expression. Which of the following is correct?

A) 12.08

B) 12.32

C) 16.08

D) 16.22

26. A cylindrical canister is 9 inches high and has a diameter of 5 inches. The formula for the volume of a cylinder is $V = \pi r^2 h$ where r is the radius and h is the height. Which of the following is the volume of the canister?

A) 176.6 in^2

B) 45 in^2

C) 141.4 in^2

D) 706.9 in^2

27. $\frac{7}{8} - \frac{1}{10} - \frac{2}{3}$

Simplify the expression. Which of the following is correct?

A) $\frac{1}{30}$

B) $\frac{13}{120}$

C) $\frac{4}{21}$

D) $\frac{4}{105}$

28. Which of the following is equivalent to $4\frac{10}{11}$?

A) 4.09

B) $4.\overline{09}$

C) 4.90

D) $4.\overline{90}$

29. Which of the following shows 74,365 rounded to the nearest hundred and to the nearest thousand?

A) hundred: 74,400; thousand: 74,000

B) hundred: 74,300; thousand: 75,000

C) hundred: 74,400; thousand: 75,000

D) hundred: 74,300; thousand: 74,000

30. A store recorded the following sales over one week:

Table 13.2. Recorded Sales

DAY	SALES
Monday	$300
Tuesday	$250
Wednesday	$550
Thursday	$475
Friday	$325
Saturday	$800

Which of the following is the ratio of the highest amount of sales to total sales for the week and the ratio of lowest amount of sales to total sales for the week?

A) lowest: $\frac{13}{108}$; highest: $\frac{8}{27}$

B) lowest: $\frac{13}{108}$; highest: $\frac{11}{54}$

C) lowest: $\frac{5}{54}$; highest: $\frac{8}{27}$

D) lowest: $\frac{5}{54}$; highest: $\frac{11}{54}$

31. $10y - 8 - 2y = 4y - 22 + 5y$

Solve the equation. Which of the following is correct?

A) $y = -4\frac{2}{3}$

B) $y = 14$

C) $y = 30$

D) $y = -30$

32. Which of the following is equivalent to 37.5%?

A) 0.0375

B) 0.375

C) 3.75

D) 37.5

33. An employee makes $37,500 per year and receives a 5.5% raise. Which of the following is the employee's new salary?

A) $35,437.50

B) $35,625

C) $39,375

D) $39,562.50

34. Which of the following sets of numbers is listed in order from least to greatest?

A) $-0.95, 0, \frac{2}{5}, 0.35, \frac{3}{4}$

B) $-1, -\frac{1}{10}, -0.11, \frac{5}{6}, 0.75$

C) $-\frac{3}{4}, -0.2, 0, \frac{2}{3}, 0.55$

D) $-1.1, -\frac{4}{5}, -0.13, 0.7, \frac{9}{11}$

35. The population of a town was 7250 in 2014 and 7375 in 2015. Which of the following was the percent increase from 2014 to 2015? (Round to the nearest tenth.)

A) 1.5%

B) 1.6%

C) 1.7%

D) 1.8%

36. Which of the following choices places these fractions in the correct order from greatest to least?

$\frac{1}{3}, -\frac{1}{4}, \frac{1}{2}, -\frac{1}{5}, \frac{1}{7}, -\frac{1}{6}$

A) $\frac{1}{2}, \frac{1}{3}, \frac{1}{7}, -\frac{1}{5}, -\frac{1}{6}, -\frac{1}{4}$

B) $\frac{1}{2}, \frac{1}{3}, \frac{1}{7}, -\frac{1}{6}, -\frac{1}{5}, -\frac{1}{4}$

C) $\frac{1}{2}, \frac{1}{7}, \frac{1}{3}, -\frac{1}{4}, -\frac{1}{5}, -\frac{1}{6}$

D) $\frac{1}{2}, \frac{1}{3}, \frac{1}{7}, -\frac{1}{6}, -\frac{1}{4}, -\frac{1}{5}$

Reading

Directions: Read the question, passage, or figure carefully, and choose the best answer.

The next three questions are based on this passage.

In its most basic form, geography is the study of space; more specifically, it studies the physical space of the earth and the ways in which it interacts with, shapes, and is shaped by its habitants. Geographers look at the world from a spatial perspective. This means that at the center of all geographic study is the question, where? For geographers, the where of any interaction, event, or development is a crucial element to understanding it.

This question of where can be asked in a variety of fields of study, so there are many sub-disciplines of geography. These can be organized into four main categories: 1) regional studies, which examine the characteristics of a particular place, 2) topical studies, which look at a single physical or human feature that impacts the whole world, 3) physical studies, which focus on the physical features of Earth, and 4) human studies, which examine the relationship between human activity and the environment.

1. A researcher studying the relationship between farming and river systems would be engaged in which of the following geographical sub-disciplines?

   A) regional studies

   B) topical studies

   C) physical studies

   D) human studies

2. Which of the following best describes the mode of the passage?

   A) expository

   B) narrative

   C) persuasive

   D) descriptive

3. Which of the following is a concise summary of the passage?

   A) The most important questions in geography are where an event or development took place.

   B) Geography, which is the study of the physical space on earth, can be broken down into four sub-disciplines.

   C) Regional studies is the study of a single region or area.

   D) Geography can be broken down into four sub-disciplines: regional studies, topical studies, physical studies, and human studies.

The next three questions are based on this passage.

It's that time again—the annual Friendswood Village Summer Fair is here! Last year we had a record number of visitors, and we're expecting an even bigger turnout this year. The fair will be bringing back all our traditional food and games, including the famous raffle. This year, we'll have a carousel, petting zoo, and climbing wall (for teenagers and adults only, please). We're also excited to welcome Petey's BBQ and Happy Tummy's Frozen Treats, who are both new to the fair this year. Tickets are available online and at local retailers.

4. Which of the following will NOT be a new presence at the Fair this year?

A) the raffle

B) the petting zoo

C) the carousel

D) Petey's BBQ

5. Based on the context, which of the following is the meaning of the word *record* in the passage?

A) a piece of evidence

B) a disk with a groove that reproduces sound

C) the best or most remarkable

D) to set down in writing

6. Which of the following best describes the mode of the passage?

A) expository

B) narrative

C) persuasive

D) descriptive

7. Based on the pattern in the headings, which of the following is a reasonable heading to insert in the blank spot?

Chapter 3. Emotions and the Central Nervous System

3A. Involuntary Physical Symptoms of Emotion

  a) Flushing

  b) _____

  c) Vocal Changes

3B. Voluntary Physical Response to Emotion

3C. Conscious Control of Emotions

A) Facial Expressions

B) Happiness

C) Emotions and Central Nervous System Disorders

D) The Cerebral Cortex

The next two questions are based on the table of contents below.

Table of Contents

3. The Cold War ....153 – 306

  A) The End of World War II ....153 – 175

  B) Escalation ....176 – 258

  C) Détente and the Final Years ....259 – 306

4. The Cold War in Popular Culture...307 – 394

  A) Contemporary Depictions of the Cold War (1945 – 1991).....307 – 363

  B) Modern Depictions of the Cold War (1992 – 2015)...........364 – 394

8. A student wants to find information on how the Potsdam Treaty, signed at the end of World War II, affected the Cold War. On which of the following pages will the student most likely find this information?

A) 155

B) 256

C) 308

D) 383

9. A researcher wants to find information on a movie made in 1967 about the Cold War. On which of the following pages should the researcher look for this information?

A) 168

B) 300

C) 311

D) 370

The next three questions are based on this passage.

Alexis de Tocqueville, a young Frenchman from an aristocratic family, visited the United States in the early 1800s. He observed: "Amongst the novel objects that attracted my attention during my stay in the United States, nothing struck me more forcibly than the general equality of conditions. [...] The more I advanced in the study of American society, the more I perceived that the equality of conditions is the fundamental fact from which all others seem to be derived, and the central point at which all my observations constantly terminated."

Excerpt from Alexis de Tocqueville's *Democracy in America*, 1835

10. Which of the following best states the main idea of the passage?

   A) Alexis de Tocqueville has contributed substantially to the study of the nineteenth-century United States.

   B) Equality was the most important ideal in the nineteenth-century United States.

   C) In nineteenth-century American society, all people had rights.

   D) American society during the nineteenth century was more equal than French society.

11. Based on the context, which of the following is the meaning of the word *novel* in the passage?

   A) new

   B) written

   C) uncertain

   D) confusing

12. The author would most likely agree with which of the following statements about the United States in the nineteenth century?

   A) Right from the beginning at least three social classes emerged, with most people falling in the middle.

   B) American people were by nature competitive and individualistic.

   C) Since the birth of the United States, its citizens have been eager to achieve and prosper.

   D) In the early decades when America had just become an independent country with a new government, people lived in equality.

13. Which of the following is an example of a primary source that would be used in a research paper on the history of mining in West Virginia?

   A) a book written by a modern historian on the growth of American unions

   B) letters written by a miner to his family in New York

   C) a recent documentary on historical mining equipment

   D) a historical novel set in a mining camp in West Virginia

14. Italics are used in the passage below for which of the following reasons?

   Spanish *conquistadors* explored what is today the Southwest United States, claiming land for Spain despite the presence of southwestern tribes.

   A) to show that a word is intentionally misspelled

   B) to indicate a word in a foreign language

   C) to emphasize a contrast

   D) to reference a footnote

15. Based on the pattern in the headings, which of the following is a reasonable heading to insert in the blank spot?

I. Types of Teas

A. Black Tea

   1) Assam

   2) Darjeeling

   3) Ceylon

B. _____

C. White Tea

A) Green Tea

B) Iced Tea

C) Cold-Brew Tea

D) Chai Tea

16. Based on the context of the passage below, which of the following is the meaning of the word *light* in the sentence?

The strange light in the room made it hard to determine the colors used in the painting.

A) a sense of mental illumination or enlightenment

B) the electromagnetic waves that make human vision possible

C) a device used to indicate right of way for traffic

D) to start a fire

The next two questions are based on this map.

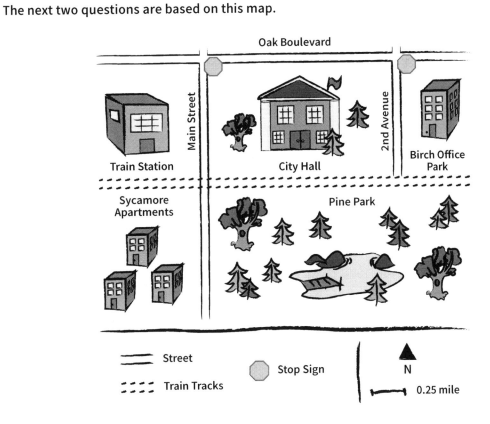

17. A family leaves the train station and heads south on Main Street. At which of the following locations will the train arrive?

A) City Hall

B) Oak Boulevard

C) Sycamore Apartments

D) Birch Office Park

18. According to the map, which of the following is the distance from City Hall to the Birch Office Park?

A) 0.1 miles

B) 1 mile

C) 10 miles

D) 100 miles

The next five questions are based on this passage.

The most important part of brewing coffee is getting the right water. Choose a water that you think has a nice, neutral flavor. Anything with too many minerals or contaminants will change the flavor of the coffee, and water with too few minerals won't do a good job of extracting the flavor from the coffee beans. Water should be heated to between 195 and 205 degrees Fahrenheit. Boiling water (212 degrees Fahrenheit) will burn the beans and give your coffee a scorched flavor.

While the water is heating, grind your beans. Remember, the fresher the grind, the fresher the flavor of the coffee. The number of beans is entirely dependent on your personal taste. Obviously, more beans will result in a more robust flavor, while fewer beans will give your coffee a more subtle taste. The texture of the grind should be not too fine (which can lead to bitter coffee) or too large (which can lead to weak coffee).

Once the beans are ground and the water has reached the perfect temperature, you're ready to brew. A French press (which we recommend), allows you to control brewing time and provide a thorough brew. Pour the grounds into the press, then pour the hot water over the grounds and let it steep. The brew shouldn't require more than 5 minutes, although those of you who like your coffee a bit harsher can leave it longer. Finally, use the plunger to remove the grounds and pour.

19. According to the passage, which of the following lists the steps for brewing coffee in the correct sequence?

   A) Choose a water that doesn't have too many or two few minerals. Then, heat water to boiling and pour over coffee grounds.

   B) Ground the beans to the appropriate texture and pour into the French press. Then, heat water to boiling and pour over the ground beans. Finally, use the plunger to remove the grounds and pour.

   C) Ground beans to the appropriate texture, and then heat water to 195 degrees Fahrenheit. Next, pour water over the grounds and steep for no more than five minutes. Finally, remove the grounds using the plunger.

   D) Choose the right type of water and heat it to the correct temperature. Next, ground the beans and put them in the French press. Then, pour the hot water over the grounds and let the coffee steep.

20. Which of the following best describes the structure of the text?

   A) chronological
   B) cause and effect
   C) problem and solution
   D) contrast

21. Which of the following statements based on the passage should be considered an opinion?

   A) While the water is heating, grind your beans.

   B) A French press (which we recommend), allows you to control brewing time and provide a thorough brew.

   C) Anything with too many minerals or contaminants will change the flavor of the coffee, and water with too few minerals won't do a good job of extracting the flavor from the coffee beans.

   D) Finally, use the plunger to remove the grounds and pour.

22. Which of the following conclusions is best supported by the passage?

   A) Coffee should never be brewed for longer than 5 minutes.

   B) It's better to use too many coffee beans when making coffee than too few.

   C) Brewing quality coffee at home is too complicated for most people to do well.

   D) The best way to brew coffee is often determined by personal preferences.

23. Which of the following would be an appropriate title for this passage?

   A) How to Brew the Perfect Cup of Coffee

   B) Why Drinking Coffee Is the Best Way to Start the Day

   C) How to Use a French Press to Make Coffee

   D) The Importance of Grinding Coffee Beans

The next two questions are based on this passage.

For an adult person to be unable to swim points to something like criminal negligence; every man, woman and child should learn. A person who cannot swim may not only become a danger to himself, but to someone, and perhaps to several, of his fellow beings. Children as early as the age of four may acquire the art; none are too young, none too old.

Frank Eugen Dalton, *Swimming Scientifically Taught*, 1912

24. Which of the following best captures the author's purpose?

   A) to encourage the reader to learn to swim

   B) to explain how people who cannot swim are a danger to others

   C) to inform the reader that it's never too late to learn to swim

   D) to argue that people who cannot swim should be punished

25. Which of the following is the purpose of this passage?

   A) to inform

   B) to entertain

   C) to describe

   D) to persuade

The next three questions are based on this passage.

NEW POLICY FOR REPLACEMENT STUDENT IDENTIFICATION CARDS

Due to recent issues with the abuse of student identification (ID) cards, Campus Security has issued a new policy for acquiring replacement student identification cards.

The following conditions must be met for students to receive a replacement student ID card:

- Student is currently enrolled in at least one class; the class may be either online or on campus.

- Student must have been issued a student ID card within the last five years.

- Student must apply for a replacement ID card in person at the Student Admissions Office. Online applications will no longer be accepted.

◆ Students will be required to pay a $25 fee for each replacement ID card. Fee may not be charged to the student's account.

Students who do not meet these conditions will be required to apply for a new ID card at the Campus Security Office.

26. Which of the following best describes the purpose of this passage?

A) to ensure that students pay the appropriate fee when applying for a replacement ID card

B) to inform students of the new policy regarding replacement ID cards

C) to inform online students that they will no longer be eligible to receive replacement ID cards

D) to punish students who have used student ID cards incorrectly in the past

27. Based on the context, which of the following is the meaning of the word *abuse* in the passage?

A) failure

B) punishment

C) misuse

D) disappearance

28. Which of the following would not be eligible to receive a replacement student ID card from the Student Admissions Office?

A) a student enrolled in one online class

B) a student who lives abroad and must apply for her replacement student ID online

C) a currently enrolled student who has lost his student ID card

D) a student who has reenrolled after a three year absence from the school

The next three questions are based on this passage.

Alfie closed his eyes and took several deep breaths. He was trying to ignore the sounds of the crowd, but even he had to admit that it was hard not to notice the tension in the stadium. He could feel 50,000 sets of eyes burning through his skin—this crowd expected perfection from him. He took another breath and opened his eyes, setting his sights on the soccer ball resting peacefully in the grass. One shot, just one last shot, between his team and the championship. He didn't look up at the goalie, who was jumping nervously on the goal line just a few yards away. Afterward, he would swear he didn't remember anything between the referee's whistle and the thunderous roar of the crowd.

29. Which of the following best describes the mode of the passage?

A) expository

B) narrative

C) persuasive

D) descriptive

30. Which of the following conclusions is best supported by the passage?

A) Alfie passed out on the field and was unable to take the shot.

B) The goalie blocked Alfie's shot.

C) Alfie scored the goal and won his team the championship.

D) The referee declared the game a tie.

31. Which of the following best describes the meaning of the phrase "he could feel 50,000 sets of eyes burning through his skin"?

A) The 50,000 people in the stadium were trying to hurt Alfie.

B) Alfie felt uncomfortable and exposed in front of my so many people.

C) Alfie felt immense pressure from the 50,000 people watching him.

D) The people in the stadium are warning Alfie that the field is on fire.

32. Which of the following indicates the beginning of a sequence?

A) Although she was initially apprehensive about the class, she soon grew to enjoy it.

B) Before he decided what to order for dinner, he had to decide on a restaurant.

C) At the moment, I can think of nothing more wonderful than a glass of lemonade.

D) To begin the restoration, they tore out the rotten floorboards.

33. Start with the shapes shown below. Follow the directions.

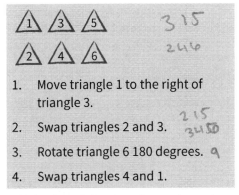

1. Move triangle 1 to the right of triangle 3.

2. Swap triangles 2 and 3.

3. Rotate triangle 6 180 degrees.

4. Swap triangles 4 and 1.

Which of the following shows the order in which the shapes now appear?

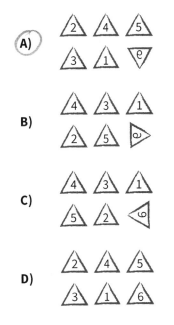

The next two questions are based on this passage.

Hannah —

Congratulations on the promotion! I just heard the news from the receptionist in Accounting—she says you're already packing up to move into your big new office.

Before you make the official move to upper management, I'd like to make sure we get proper documentation in place for your replacement. (You remember what a pain it was when you trained a few years ago.) To that end, could you please make a list of your current job responsibilities and include a list of all currently available training material that will be necessary for the person who takes over that job? If you feel new training documents are necessary, please include a description of these, and I'll have someone type them up for you.

Congratulations again—you've earned it.

Best regards,

Sasha

34. Which of the following best captures the author's purpose?

A) to inform Hannah that the receptionist in Accounting is telling people about her promotion

B) to let Hannah know she has performed well at work despite not receiving good training

C) to congratulate Hannah on her promotion

D) to acquire information from Hannah in order to train her replacement

35. Which of the following best describes the relationship of the writer to Hannah?

A) Hannah's manager

B) Hannah's coworker

C) Hannah's friend

D) Hannah's replacement

The next two questions are based on the passage below.

East River High School has released its graduation summary for the class of 2016. Out of a total of 558 senior students, 525 (94 percent) successfully completed their degree program and graduated. Of these, 402 (representing 72 percent of the total class) went on to attend to a two- or four-year college or university. The distribution of students among the four main types of colleges and universities—small or large private and small or large public—is shown in the figure below. As the data shows, the majority of East River High School's college-attending graduates chose a large, public institution.

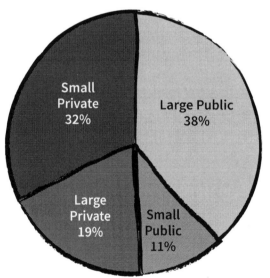

36. According to the figure, how many students from East River High School will attend a small, public college or university?

A) 4

B) 44

C) 440

D) 4400

37. Which of the following best describes the tone of the passage?

A) professional

B) casual

C) concerned

D) congratulatory

38. A man is examining cake recipes to find one that will be suitable for his friend, who cannot eat dairy products. According the lists of required ingredients, which of the following should he choose?

A) Recipe Ingredients – flour, sugar, water, milk, eggs, baking powder, baking soda, chocolate powder, almonds

B) Recipe Ingredients – cake flour, vegetable oil, butter, eggs, baking powder, chocolate chips

C) Recipe Ingredients – flour, brown sugar, butter, eggs, baking soda, vanilla extract, macadamia nuts

D) Recipe Ingredients – flour, sugar, brown sugar, vegetable oil, eggs, applesauce, baking powder, vanilla extract

39. A student has written the paragraph below as an introduction to a paper. Which of the following is most likely the topic of the paper?

> It has now been two decades since the introduction of thermonuclear fusion weapons into the military inventories of the great powers, and more than a decade since the United States, Great Britain, and the Soviet Union ceased to test nuclear weapons in the atmosphere. Today our understanding of the technology of thermonuclear weapons seems highly advanced, but our knowledge of the physical and biological consequences of nuclear war is continuously evolving.
>
> United States Arms Control and Disarmament Agency, Worldwide Effects of Nuclear War: Some Perspectives, 1998

A) the impact of thermonuclear weapons on the military

B) the technology of thermonuclear weapons

C) atmospheric testing of nuclear weapons

D) the physical and biological consequences of nuclear war

The next two questions are based on this passage.

Ms. Rodriguez —

A recent review of our accounts has shown that you were mistakenly overcharged for your October water bill. Due to a system error, customers in your area were charged twice for their October water usage. We regret the error, and are currently in the process of issuing refunds using the following criteria:

- Customers who paid with a debit card or bank account will receive refunds directly deposited into their bank accounts.
- Credit card transactions will be canceled by our company and will not appear on your statement.
- Customer who paid via check will receive a refund check in the mail in 4 – 6 weeks.

Your business is important to us, and we value your continued support. To demonstrate our commitment to our customers, we will be offering a 5% discount during the month of November to customers affected by this accounting error.

Please contact me directly if you have any questions about your bill or the refund process.

Regards,

Timothy Halgren

Director, Customer Relations

Greenway Water Company

40. Which of the following best describes the purpose of the passage?

A) to inform customers that they will receive a 5% discount on their water bills during the month of November

B) to inform customers that they were overcharged and will be receiving refunds

C) to urge customers to contact their customer service representatives with questions about their bills

D) to thank customers for their continued support

41. Which of the following conclusions is well supported by the passage?

A) Greenway Water Company will soon go out of business when customers leave.

B) Ms. Rodriguez will receive a refund check in the mail in 4 – 6 weeks.

C) Greenway Water Company is concerned that customers may be upset by the error.

D) All customers of Greenway Water Company will receive refunds for being overcharged in October.

The next two questions are based on the index below.

New Zealand ....125 – 127, 212 – 215, 306

Nicaragua .... 76, 132 – 151

Niger .... 15 – 22, 317 – 320

Nigeria... 16 – 18, 246

North Korea ....101 – 105, 221 – 231, 313

Norway... 135 – 140, 295

42. A student wants to find information on the Oslo, the capital of Norway. According the index for a geography book, where should the student look first?

A) 15

B) 125

C) 135

D) 221

43. A student wants to find information on rivers in Niger. According the index for a geography book, where should the student look first?

A) 15

B) 101

C) 212

D) 313

The next three questions are based on this passage.

We've been told for years that the recipe for weight loss is fewer calories in than calories out. In other words, eat less and exercise more, and your body will take care of the rest. As many of those who've tried to diet can attest, this edict doesn't always produce results. If you're one of those folks, you might have felt that you just weren't doing it right—that the failure was all your fault.

However, several new studies released this year have suggested that it might not be your fault at all. For example, a study of people who'd lost a high percentage of their body weight (>17%) in a short period of time found that they could not physically maintain their new weight. Scientists measured their resting metabolic rate and found that they'd need to consume only a few hundred calories a day to meet their metabolic needs. Basically, their bodies were in starvation mode and seemed to desperately hang on to each and every calorie. Eating even a single healthy, well-balanced meal a day would cause these subjects to start packing back on the pounds.

Other studies have shown that factors like intestinal bacteria, distribution of body fat, and hormone levels can affect the manner in which our bodies process calories. There's also the fact that it's actually quite difficult to measure the number of calories consumed during a particular meal and the number used while exercising.

44. Which of the following would be the best summary statement to conclude the passage?

   A) It turns out that conventional dieting wisdom doesn't capture the whole picture of how our bodies function.

   B) Still, counting calories and tracking exercise is a good idea if you want to lose weight.

   C) In conclusion, it's important to lose weight responsibly: losing too much weight at once can negatively impact the body.

   D) It's easy to see that diets don't work, so we should focus less on weight loss and more on overall health.

45. Which of the following type of arguments is used in the passage?

   A) emotional argument

   B) appeal to authority

   C) specific evidence

   D) rhetorical questioning

46. Which of the following would weaken the author's argument?

   A) a new diet pill from a pharmaceutical company that promises to help patients lose weight by changing intestinal bacteria

   B) the personal experience of a man who was able to lose a significant amount of weight taking in fewer calories than he used

   C) a study showing that people in different geographic locations lose different amounts of weight when on the same diet

   D) a study showing that people often misreport their food intake when part of a scientific study on weight loss

The next two questions are based on this chart.

Table 13.3. Prices of Office Supplies

MANUFACTURER	SHIPPING AND HANDLING
Discount Office Supplies	$0.99 per pound
Paper Clips & Staples	$12.99 flat fee for all packages
Quick & Fast Office Supplies	$7.99 flat fee for all packages under 10 pounds; $1.99 per additional pound
Blanchard Supplies	free shipping on packages under 10 pounds; $15.99 flat fee for all packages over 10 pounds

47. A company is planning ordering office supplies that will weigh 22 pounds. Based on the pricing chart, which of the following manufacturers would offer the lowest cost for shipping and handling?

   A) Discount Office Supplies

   B) Paper Clips & Staples

   C) Quick & Fast Office Supplies

   D) Blanchard Supplies

48. A company is placing an order for office supplies that will weigh 11 pounds. Based on the pricing chart, which of the following manufacturers would offer the lowest cost for shipping and handling?

   A) Discount Office Supplies

   B) Paper Clips & Staples

   C) Quick & Fast Office Supplies

   D) Blanchard Supplies

The next two questions are based on this passage.

American Cowslip: This plant grows spontaneously in Virginia and other parts of North America. It flowers in the beginning of May, and the seeds ripen in July, soon after which the stalks and leaves decay, so that the roots remain inactive till the following spring. It is propagated by offsets, which the roots put out freely when they are in a loose moist soil and a shady situation; the best time to remove the roots, and take away the offsets, is in August, after the leaves and stalks are decayed, that they may be fixed well in their new situation before the frost comes on.

William Curtis, *The Botanical Magazine*, 1790

49. According to the passage, which of the following is the best time to remove the roots of American Cowslip?

   A) August

   B) May

   C) July

   D) December

50. Which of the following is the meaning of *propagated* as used in the sentence?

   A) killed

   B) multiplied

   C) extracted

   D) concealed

51. According to the figure below, which of the following is a difference between pyrimidine and purine bases?

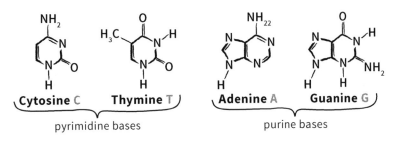

Cytosine C   Thymine T

pyrimidine bases

Adenine A   Guanine G

purine bases

- **A)** Pyrimidine bases do not include an amine group (NH_2), while purine bases do.
- **B)** Pyrimidine bases have an oxygen atom, while purine bases do not.
- **C)** Pyrimidine bases have a single carbon nitrogen ring, while purine bases have two.
- **D)** Pyrimidine bases are found in DNA and RNA, while purine bases are found only in DNA.

52. Which of the following represents the temperature in degrees Fahrenheit according to the thermometer above?

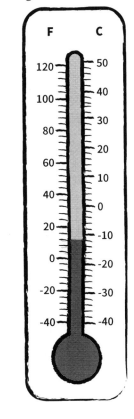

- **A)** −10
- **B)** 48
- **C)** 54
- **D)** 76

53. Based on the pattern in the headings, which of the following is a reasonable heading to insert in the blank spot?

5. The Human Digestive System

A. The Digestive Tract
    1) Mouth
    2) Esophagus
    3) _____
    4) Intestines

B. Accessory Organs
    1) Salivary Glands
    2) Liver
    3) Gall Bladder

- **A)** Stomach
- **B)** Pancreas
- **C)** Heart
- **D)** Proteins

Science

Directions: Read the question carefully, and choose the best answer.

1. The process by which blood circulates oxygen from the lungs to the body's tissues is an example of which of the following?

    A) external respiration

    B) internal respiration

    C) inhalation

    D) exhalation

2. Which of the following is the material that is secreted into hair follicles to waterproof and lubricate the skin?

    A) sweat

    B) sebum

    C) vernix caseosa

    D) mucus

3. Which of the following are the connective tissues that attach bone to bone and help strengthen joints?

    A) tendons

    B) cartilage

    C) collagen

    D) ligaments

4. Which of the following is NOT a nucleobase of DNA?

    A) adenine

    B) guanine

    C) thymine

    D) uracil

5. Which of the following materials is the primary structural protein of the epidermis, nails, and skin?

    A) eponychium

    B) collagen

    C) keratin

    D) fibroblast

6. Which of the following correctly describes atomic number?

    A) The atomic number is the number of atoms in a mole of a given substance.

    B) The atomic number is the number of neutrons in an atom.

    C) The atomic number is the number of atoms in a gram of a given substance.

    D) The atomic number is the number of protons in an atom.

7. Which of the following is a descriptive, generalized body of scientific observations?

    A) law

    B) theory

    C) model

    D) hypothesis

8. Which of the following types of cells are the main transporters of oxygen through the body?

    A) goblet cells

    B) white blood cells

    C) red blood cells

    D) platelets

9. Which of the following is the general term for a chemical substance that the body produces and transports through the blood to stimulate a cellular response?

    A) hypophysis

    B) amino acids

    C) oxytocin

    D) hormones

10. Which of the following is NOT a function of hair?

   A) regulation of body temperature
   B) extension of the sensory system
   C) protection from UV radiation
   D) protecting soft tissue from injury

11. Which of the following is NOT one of the functions of proteins found in the phospholipid bilayer of a cell membrane?

   A) to break down material that enters through the cell membrane
   B) to act as receptors that recognize and transmit hormonal messages
   C) to provide an attachment point for other cells
   D) to transport material across the membrane into the cell

12. Which of the following is the muscular action that moves a part of the body away from its median plane?

   A) abduction
   B) adduction
   C) pronation
   D) supination

13. Which of the following does NOT distinguish quantitative data collection from qualitative data collection methods?

   A) Qualitative methods are more open-ended than quantitative.
   B) Results from randomized quantitative methods can be applied to a general population; results from qualitative cannot.
   C) Quantitative methods are number based; qualitative methods are text based.
   D) Qualitative methods do not need to be as valid or reliable as quantitative methods.

14. Which of the following is an example of a birthmark caused by an increased volume of capillaries close to the surface of the skin?

   A) ephelides
   B) vascular nevis
   C) melanocytes
   D) comedones

15. Which of the following correctly describes the valence shell of an atom?

   A) The valence shell is the outermost-occupied electron orbital energy level.
   B) The valence shell is always partially filled with electrons.
   C) The valence shell is found only in ions, not in neutral atoms.
   D) The valence shell must contain p-orbitals.

16. Which of the following describes how skeletal muscles and bones work together to stimulate movement?

   A) Muscles contract and exert force on the bone, which acts as a lever to stimulate movement.
   B) Bones contract and exert force on the muscle, which acts as a lever to stimulate movement.
   C) Muscles elongate, moving the bone involuntarily.
   D) Bones elongate, moving the muscle involuntarily.

17. Which of the following describes the correct order of stages of the cell cycle?

   A) interphase → mitosis → cytokinesis
   B) prophase → metaphase → anaphase → telophase
   C) interphase → meiosis I → meiosis II
   D) gap I → synthesis → gap II

18. Which of the following occurs due to a hypersensitivity in the immune system that causes a major inflammatory response to a common material?

    A) development of antibodies

    B) autoimmune disorders

    C) allergies

    D) AIDS

19. Which of the following is one of the primary muscles that drives ventilation?

    A) thoracic cavity

    B) oblique

    C) lungs

    D) diaphragm

20. White blood cells develop from stem cells located in which of the following organs?

    A) thymus

    B) bone marrow

    C) lymph node

    D) spleen

21. Which of the following describes a gene in which one allele takes a different form from another?

    A) phenotype

    B) heterozygous

    C) homolog

    D) homozygous

22. Which of the following are the two proteins found in muscle tissue that cause muscle contraction as they slide past one another?

    A) actin and sarcomeres

    B) actin and myosin

    C) myosin and tropomyosin

    D) troponin and sarcomeres

23. Which of the following molecules have London dispersion forces?

    A) All atoms and molecules have London dispersion forces.

    B) Atoms and molecules with full valence shells have London dispersion forces.

    C) Atoms and molecules with a noble gas electron configuration have London dispersion forces.

    D) Atoms and molecules that contain at least one metal atom have London dispersion forces.

24. Which of the following is NOT a hormone-producing gland of the endocrine system?

    A) steroid

    B) pituitary

    C) adrenal

    D) thyroid

25. Which of the following is the process in which pathogens are "eaten," or absorbed and digested, by white blood cells as part of an immune response?

    A) pinocytosis

    B) phagocytosis

    C) opsonization

    D) vasodilation

26. Which of the following describes the relationship between correlation and causation?

    A) Correlation implies causation.

    B) Only negative correlation implies causation.

    C) Correlation and causation are mutually exclusive; if one happens, the other cannot.

    D) Correlation does not imply causation.

27. The exchange of gases and blood happens in which of the following parts of the respiratory zone?

   A) alveoli

   B) alveolar duct

   C) pleura

   D) bronchioles

28. Which of the following glands provides nourishment for sperm, as well as the majority of the fluid that combines with sperm to form semen?

   A) seminal vesicles

   B) prostate gland

   C) bulbourethral glands

   D) Cowper's glands

29. Which of the following is the largest branch of the abdominal aorta, which supplies oxygenated blood to the upper digestive tract?

   A) inferior mesenteric artery

   B) gastric artery

   C) celiac artery

   D) superior mesenteric artery

30. Which of the following is NOT a phase of spermatogenesis, or the final stage of sperm formation?

   A) tail formation

   B) cap phase

   C) Golgi phase

   D) fertilization

31. Blood is metabolized in the liver as it passes through which of the following types of blood vessels?

   A) hepatic vein

   B) inferior vena cava

   C) arterioles

   D) sinusoidal capillaries

32. Which of the following is a heterogeneous mixture?

   A) a mixture in which the atoms or molecules are distributed unevenly

   B) a mixture of more than one type of atom or molecule

   C) a mixture of covalent and ionic compounds

   D) a mixture of polar and nonpolar molecules

33. Hormones can be classified into one of four basic groups based on their chemical source. Which of the following groups is derived from cholesterol?

   A) catecholamines

   B) steroids

   C) polypeptides

   D) eicosanoids

34. Which of the following is a definition of adaptation, in the context of evolution?

   A) the process of descent with modification

   B) the increased likelihood that a particular genotype will increase in frequency in a population

   C) the process of individuals in a population choosing mates due to superior characteristics

   D) a biological feature or behavior in a population of organisms that improves its chances for survival in the environment

35. Which of the following is the element of blood that comprises most of its total volume?

   A) plasma

   B) red blood cells

   C) white blood cells

   D) water

36. Which of the following is NOT true for enzyme-catalyzed reactions?

A) The reaction will speed up if the concentration of substrate increases.

B) The reaction will speed up if the concentration of enzyme increases.

C) The reaction will slow down at very low temperatures.

D) The reaction will speed up without limit as the temperature increases.

37. Which of the following is the molecule found in red blood cells that binds to up to four oxygen molecules?

A) hemoglobin

B) erythrocytes

C) globulin

D) antigens

38. Which of the following is NOT a reason why randomization is critical in experimental design, especially in experiments with human subjects?

A) to give humans no choice but to participate

B) to eliminate selection bias

C) to provide a statistical basis

D) to provide a balanced group of subjects

39. Which of the following is the division of the nervous system primarily responsible for regulating all involuntary and subconscious muscle functions?

A) somatic nervous system

B) autonomic nervous system

C) sympathetic nervous system

D) peripheral nervous system

40. Which of the following is an appendage of a neuron that sends electrical signals away from the neuron cell?

A) axon

B) dendrite

C) neurite

D) neuroglia

41. Which of the following is the definition of action potential in a neuron?

A) a connection between two neurons

B) an electrical impulse that is transported down a neuron in response to a stimulus

C) an imbalanced electrical charge that exists in an inactive nerve cell

D) a chemical signal between two nerve cells

42. Which of the following are the three major portions of the brain?

A) cerebellum, spinal cord, white matter

B) cerebrum, temporal lobe, occipital lobe

C) pons, medulla oblongata, brain stem

D) cerebrum, cerebellum, brain stem

43. Which of the following describes how a catalyst speeds up a reaction?

A) A catalyst participates in the reaction, making it go faster.

B) A catalyst speeds up a reaction by causing lower energy products to be made.

C) A catalyst lowers the activation energy by providing an alternate route for the reaction.

D) A catalyst causes the reactants to collide more frequently.

44. Which of the following is the final vessel through which semen must pass before being expelled from the body?

A) ejaculatory duct

B) penile urethra

C) membranous urethra

D) vas deferens

45. Which of the following groups of bones are part of the axial skeleton?

A) pectoral girdle

B) rib cage

C) arms and hands

D) pelvic girdle

46. Which of the following types of variables is changed in a scientific experiment?

A) controlled variable

B) measured variable

C) dependent variable

D) independent variable

47. The vertebral column consists of thirty-three vertebrae and is divided into several groups. Which of the following describes the lumbar vertebrae?

A) seven vertebrae located in the neck that connect the vertebral column to the skull, allowing for neck rotation

B) five vertebrae that are fused in the pelvis, forming a supportive, wedge-shaped bone

C) twelve vertebrae located in the upper back, each of which connects to the base of a rib

D) five vertebrae located in the lower back, which support most of the body's weight

48. Which type of hypothesis assumes no relationship between two variables?

A) scientific hypothesis

B) working hypothesis

C) null hypothesis

D) alternate hypothesis

49. Which of the following describes the applicability of a research conclusion to situations outside the experiment?

A) internal validity

B) test validity

C) external validity

D) content validity

50. Which of the following is NOT one of the three types of muscles found in the human body?

A) skeletal

B) cardiac

C) soft

D) smooth

51. Which of the following is the structure of the male reproductive system that stores spermatozoa during the maturation process?

A) vas deferens

B) scrotum

C) epididymis

D) testicular artery

52. Which of the following types of hormones stimulates a chemical response to a target cell by diffusing through the cell membrane to bind to the receptors inside the cell?

A) fat-soluble hormones

B) amino acid derivatives

C) hydrophilic hormones

D) water-soluble hormones

53. Which of the following is an example of human error in an experiment?

A) an imperfectly calibrated scale

B) contaminating a sterile sample by breathing on it

C) a draft in the laboratory slightly changing the temperature of a liquid

D) failure to account for wind speed when measuring distance traveled

English and Language Arts

Directions: Read the question carefully, and choose the best answer.

1. *Cats* is italicized for which of the following reasons?

   > In 1983, almost twenty years after his death, T.S. Eliot won two Tony Awards for his contributions to the well-loved musical *Cats*.

   A) to highlight its importance

   B) to indicate it is intentionally misspelled

   C) because it is the title of a musical

   D) because it is in a foreign language

2. Which of the following phrases contains an error in capitalization?

   > The *Chicago Tribune* is famous for many reasons: in 1948, the paper published an erroneous headline about the winner of the Presidential election, and in 1974, it called for President Nixon's resignation.

   A) *Chicago Tribune*

   B) the paper

   C) Presidential election

   D) President Nixon's

3. Which of the following punctuation marks correctly completes the sentence?

   > In the eighteenth century, renowned composer Wolfgang Amadeus Mozart set to music the poetry of a famous, well-known writer who shared his name_Johann Wolfgang von Goethe.

   A) ,

   B) :

   C) ;

   D) ?

4. Which of the following sentences has the correct subject-verb agreement?

   A) The Iris and B. Gerald Cantor Roof Garden, atop the Metropolitan Museum of Art in New York City, offer a remarkable view.

   B) The Mammoth-Flint Ridge Cave System, located in central Kentucky inside Mammoth Cave National Park, are the largest cave system in the world.

   C) Andy Warhol's paintings, in addition to being the subject of the largest single-artist museum in the United States, are in great demand.

   D) The field of child development are concerned with the emotional, psychological, and biological developments of infants and children.

5. Which of the following would most likely be found in a scientific paper on the history of telescopes?

   A) Jerry R. Ehman had always encouraged his kids' love of science by taking them camping and star gazing.

   B) In 1977, Jerry R. Ehman, using a powerful radio telescope, detected a signal that seemed to come from outside the Earth's atmosphere.

   C) I believe that telescopes have the potential to change our understanding of the universe and our place in it.

   D) It's really silly to think that telescopes are a new invention.

6. Which of the following is part of the predicate in the sentence?

> Vivariums, common in elementary school classrooms, are enclosed spaces designed to replicate a particular habitat.

A) are enclosed spaces

B) vivariums

C) elementary school classrooms

D) common in

7. Which of the following is misspelled in the sentence?

> The Boat Race, a rowing race that has been held almost annually in London, England, since 1856, was infamously interupted in 2012.

A) rowing

B) annually

C) infamously

D) interupted

8. Which of the following is misspelled in the sentence?

> The exotic pet trade is a significant concern for enviornmentalists and animal rights advocates around the world.

A) significant

B) enviornmentalists

C) rights

D) advocates

9. Which of the following is a synonym for *standardized* as used in the sentence?

> In baseball today, strict regulations have standardized the design of bats; they used to come in a wide range of shapes, sizes, and weights.

A) clarified

B) reconciled

C) normalized

D) ignored

10. Which of the following prefixes would be used to indicate that something is opposite?

A) fore–

B) bi–

C) anti–

D) trans–

11. Which of the following sentences has correct pronoun-antecedent agreement?

A) Animals use estivation to avoid harsh conditions and to help it survive winter.

B) Some species of fish use luminescent lures to trick other fish into moving closer to it.

C) In a parasitic relationship, one species is negatively affected while the other species acquires what they need to survive.

D) Tropical rainforests are made up of many layers, each of which has its own distinct species.

12. Which of the following is an appropriate synonym for *insolent* as it is used in the sentence?

> The students' insolent behavior drove the teacher to punish the class with extra homework.

A) confusing

B) disrespectful

C) delightful

D) unlikely

13. Which of the following root words would be used in a word related to time?

A) gram

B) crypt

C) chron

D) mort

14. Which of the following is correctly punctuated?

A) In addition to the disastrous effects an active volcano can have on it's immediate surroundings, an eruption can also pose a threat to passing aircraft.

B) In addition to the disastrous effects an active volcano can have on it's immediate surroundings: an eruption can also pose a threat to passing aircraft.

C) In addition to the disastrous effects an active volcano can have on its immediate surroundings: an eruption can also pose a threat to passing aircraft.

D) In addition to the disastrous effects an active volcano can have on its immediate surroundings, an eruption can also pose a threat to passing aircraft.

15. Which of the following would be an acceptable way to combine the two clauses?

A) While these incidents sometimes end in funny or heartwarming stories, at other times they end in fear and destruction.

B) While these incidents sometimes end in funny or heartwarming stories; at other times they end in fear and destruction.

C) While these incidents sometimes end in funny or heartwarming stories: at other times they end in fear and destruction.

D) While these incidents sometimes end in funny or heartwarming stories—at other times they end in fear and destruction.

16. Which of the following is an appropriate synonym for *advancing* as it is used in the sentence?

L.L. Zamenhof, an ophthalmologist in the late 1800s, invented a universal language called Esperanto with the goal of advancing international communications and relations.

A) improving

B) changing

C) hastening

D) celebrating

17. Which of the following is a simple sentence?

A) Although Sacagawea is famous for her role as guide and interpreter for Lewis and Clark, few know about the mystery surrounding her death.

B) The high death toll at the end of the Civil War was not exclusively due to battle losses; large numbers of soldiers died as a result of poor living conditions.

C) Self-driving vehicles are just now being introduced on the automotive market, but research into automating vehicle processes began as early as the 1920s.

D) Freediving is sometimes combined with other underwater activities such as photography, football, hockey, and even target shooting.

18. In the sentence, the prefix *lexi–* indicates that the researcher studies which of the following?

The distinguished lexicologist had been with the university for many years.

A) literature

B) words

C) plants

D) rocks

19. Which of the following is a complex sentence?

A) Engineers designed seat belts to stop the inertia of traveling bodies by applying an opposing force to the driver and passengers during a collision.

B) Hurricanes cost the United States roughly $5 billion per year in damages and have been the cause of almost two million deaths in the last two hundred years.

C) Woodstock appeared in the *Peanuts* comic strips as early as April of 1967, but he was not named until June of 1970, ten months after the famous music festival of the same name, Woodstock.

D) Although organized firefighting groups existed as early as ancient Egyptian times, the first fully state-run brigade was created by Emperor Augustus of Rome.

20. Which of the following sentences is irrelevant as part of a paragraph composed of these sentences?

A) It looks like the weather might force us to move the game to next weekend.

B) Our team will be playing our biggest rival for the last game of the season.

C) The teams play each other every year, and it's a big event for the town.

D) Last year, the mayor closed down Main Street so fans could celebrate together safely.

21. According to Greek mythology, Narcissus was a hunter who was so handsome that he fell in love with his own reflection.

Which of the following parts of speech is *handsome* as it is used in the sentence?

A) noun

B) verb

C) adjective

D) adverb

22. Which of the following words from the sentence is slang?

It's a drag to do homework on the weekend, but I won't pass the class if I spend all day watching TV.

A) homework

B) pass

C) spend

D) drag

23. Which of the following punctuation marks is used incorrectly?

In many European countries such as, France, Spain, and Italy, hot chocolate is made with real melted chocolate making for a beverage that is thick and rich.

A) the comma after "as"

B) the comma after "France"

C) the comma after "Italy"

D) the period after "rich"

24. Which of the following nouns is written in the correct plural form?

A) shelves

B) phenomenons

C) mans

D) deers

25. Which of the following parts of speech is *travels* as used in the sentence?

> Abby's travels in Asia provided her the opportunity to try many foods that she would not have been able to try at home in the United States.

A) verb

B) noun

C) adjective

D) adverb

26. Which of the following punctuation marks is used incorrectly?

> Although the Nile River in Africa, passes through eleven countries, it is the main water source of only two of them—Egypt and Sudan.

A) the comma after *Africa*

B) the comma after *countries*

C) the em-dash after *them*

D) the period after *Sudan*

27. Which is the best way to revise the underlined portion of the sentences?

> Spelunking involves much more than adrenaline: enthusiasts dive into unexplored caves <u>to study structures of, take photographs, and create maps of</u> the untouched systems.

A) to study structures of, take photographs, and create maps of

B) to study structures of, to take photographs, and create maps of

C) to study structures of, taking photographs of, and creating maps of

D) to study structures, take photographs, and create maps of

28.

Table 13.4. Outline

I. The Stages of Labor
  A) First Stage
    1. Early Phase
    2. Active Phase
    3. Transition Phase
  B) Second Stage
    1. Pushing
    2. Fetal Expulsion
  C) Third Stage
  D) Fourth Stage

Which of the following statements is true regarding the outline?

A) The Fourth Stage of labor is broken down into two phases.

B) The First Stage of labor is the longest.

C) The First Stage of labor is broken into three phases.

D) Pushing and Fetal Expulsion are parts of the Third Stage of labor.

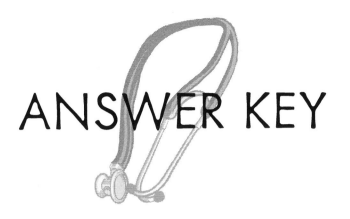

ANSWER KEY

Mathematics

1. **D)**

Substitute 5 for x:

$4(5) \div (5 - 1) = 20 \div 4 = 5$

2. **C)**

The slope of a horizontal line is zero because the change in y is zero.

3. **C)**

Alex and David split an appetizer that costs $8.50, so each will pay $4.25 in addition to the price of the entrée. Rachel orders an appetizer for $6.50, plus lemonade for $3, so she will pay $9.50 in addition to the price of the entrée.

$9.50 - $4.25 = $5.25

4. **B)**

Subtract the percentage of boys from 100% to find the percentage of girls:

$100\% - 46\% = 54\%$

Find 21% of 54% of 450:

$0.21 \times 0.54 \times 450 \approx 51$

5. **C)**

First convert 15,140 drops to seconds using the ratio given:

$15{,}140 \text{ drops} \times \frac{4 \text{ sec.}}{1 \text{ drop}} = 60{,}560 \text{ sec.}$

Now convert seconds to hours:

$60{,}560 \text{ sec.} \times \frac{1 \text{ min.}}{60 \text{ sec.}} \times \frac{1 \text{ hr.}}{60 \text{ min.}} = 16.8\overline{2} \text{ hr.}$

Convert the remainder of hours back to minutes and seconds:

$0.8\overline{2} \text{ hr.} \times \frac{60 \text{ min.}}{1 \text{ hr.}} = 49.\overline{3} \text{ min.}$

$0.\overline{3} \text{ min.} \times \frac{60 \text{ sec}}{1 \text{ min.}} = 20 \text{ sec.}$

16 hours, 49 minutes, 20 seconds

6. **D)**

First complete the operations in parentheses: $(3 + 5)^2 + 24 \div 16 - 5 \div 2 = (8)^2 + 24 \div 16 - 5 \div 2$

Next solve the exponents: $(8)^2 + 24 \div 16 - 5 \div 2 = 64 + 24 \div 16 - 5 \div 2$

Then complete multiplication and division operations: $64 + 24 \div 16 - 5 \div 2 = 64 + 1.5 - 2.5$

Finally complete addition and subtraction operations: $64 + 1.5 - 2.5 = 63$

7. **C)**

First convert the length of the race to miles:

$10 \text{ km} \times \frac{1000 \text{ m}}{1 \text{ km}} \times \frac{1 \text{ ft.}}{0.3048 \text{ m}} \times \frac{1 \text{ mi.}}{5280 \text{ ft.}} = 6.21 \text{ mi.}$

Next convert her training pace to minutes (in decimal form):

$15 \text{ sec.} \times \frac{1 \text{ min.}}{60 \text{ sec.}} = 0.25 \text{ min.}$

8 min., 15 sec. = 8 min. + 0.25 min. = 8.25 min.

Then multiply the length of the race by her pace per mile:

6.21 mi. × $\frac{8.25 \text{ min.}}{1 \text{ mi.}}$ = 51.23 min.

Finally convert the time back to min:sec form:

0.23 min. × $\frac{60 \text{ sec.}}{1 \text{ min.}}$ = 14 sec.

51:14

8. D)

Flip the divisor fraction and multiply:

$\frac{8}{15} \div \frac{1}{6} = \frac{8}{15} \times \frac{6}{1} = \frac{8 \times 6}{15 \times 1} = \frac{48}{15}$

Then reduce the fraction by dividing numerator and denominator by the greatest common factor:

$\frac{48}{15} = \frac{48 \div 3}{15 \div 3} = \frac{16}{5}$

Finally divide the whole numbers to find the mixed fraction:

$\frac{16}{5} = 3\frac{1}{5}$

9. A)

$5\frac{1}{3}$ tbsp. of lemon juice should be used.

Set up a ratio:

$\frac{2 \text{ tbsp.}}{\frac{1}{4} \text{ c.}} = \frac{x}{\frac{2}{3} \text{ c.}}$

Now cross-multiply:

$(2 \text{ tbsp.})\left(\frac{2}{3} \text{ c.}\right) = (x)\left(\frac{1}{4} \text{ c.}\right)$

$x = \frac{(2 \text{ tbsp.})\left(\frac{2}{3} \text{ c.}\right)}{\frac{1}{4} \text{ c.}} = 5\frac{1}{3}$ tbsp.

10. C)

$x = \frac{\text{female 9th graders}}{\text{total 9th graders}}$ and

$y = \frac{\text{total 9th graders}}{\text{total students}}$

You are looking for the proportion $\frac{\text{female 9th graders}}{\text{total students}}$. See that multiplying x by y cancels out "total 9th graders" in the numerator and denominator and gives this proportion:

$x \times y = \frac{\text{female 9th graders}}{\text{total 9th graders}} \times \frac{\text{total 9th graders}}{\text{total students}}$

$= \frac{\text{female 9th graders}}{\text{total students}}$

11. A)

First calculate his original weekly work hours:

$\frac{8 \text{ hr.}}{1 \text{ day}} \times \frac{5 \text{ days}}{1 \text{ wk.}} = \frac{40 \text{ hr.}}{\text{wk.}}$

Next calculate his current weekly work hours:

$\frac{8 \text{ hr.}}{1 \text{ day}} \times \frac{3 \text{ days}}{1 \text{ wk.}} + \frac{4 \text{ hr.}}{1 \text{ day}} \times \frac{2 \text{ days}}{1 \text{ wk.}} = \frac{32 \text{ hr.}}{\text{wk.}}$

Now find the difference in hours and divide by his original hours to find the percentage change:

$\frac{40 \text{ hr./wk.} - 32 \text{ hr./wk.}}{40 \text{ hr./wk.}} = \frac{x}{100}$

$(8 \text{ hr./wk.})(100) = (40 \text{ hr./wk.})(x)$

$x = \frac{(8 \text{ hr./wk.})(100)}{(40 \text{ hr./wk.})} = 20$

Toledo's weekly work hours have decreased by 20%.

12. A)

Convert fractions to a common denominator and compare numerators:

$\frac{2}{16} = \frac{6}{48}$

$\frac{1}{24} = \frac{2}{48}$

$\frac{3}{32} = \frac{4.5}{48}$

$\frac{3}{16} = \frac{9}{48}$

$\frac{2}{48} < \frac{4.5}{48} < \frac{5}{48} < \frac{6}{48} < \frac{9}{48}$

13. A)

First subtract 4 from both sides:

$3a + 4 - 4 = 2a - 4$

$3a = 2a - 4$

Next subtract $2a$ from both sides (remember that the minus sign remains before the 4):

$3a - 2a = 2a - 4 - 2a$

$a = -4$

14. D)

A proportion is written using two ratios relating pages to minutes, with x representing the number of unknown minutes: $\frac{40}{45} = \frac{265}{x}$. The proportion is solved by cross-multiplying and dividing: $40x = 11{,}925$, $x = 298.125$. The solution is approximately 298 minutes.

15. **D)**

The money Jane earns is equal to $15 times the number of hours she babysits:

$15h$

The total money in Jane's bank account is equal to the money she started with plus the money she earns:

$275 + 15h$

Set this expression equal to $400:

$400 = 275 + 15h$

16. **C)**

This rectangular prism has 2 sides that are 12 inches by 18 inches, 2 sides that are 12 inches by 6 inches, and 2 sides that are 18 inches by 6 inches. Add the area of all the sides to find the total surface area:

$SA = 2lw + 2lh + 2wh$

$SA = 2(12 \text{ in.})(18 \text{ in.}) + 2(12 \text{ in.})(6 \text{ in.}) + 2(18 \text{ in.})(6 \text{ in.})$

$SA = 432 \text{ in.}^2 + 144 \text{ in.}^2 + 216 \text{ in.}^2 = 792 \text{ in.}^2$

17. **C)**

The answer choices are 24, −2, 30, and 0 for A, B, C, and D, respectively. Answer choice C, 30, is the greatest value for all of the responses.

18. **B)**

First find the radius of the pizza:

$r = \dfrac{d}{2}$

$r = \dfrac{10 \text{ in.}}{2} = 5 \text{ in.}$

Next use the formula for sector area:

$A = \pi r^2 \dfrac{\theta}{360°}$

$A = \pi (5 \text{ in.})^2 \dfrac{40°}{360°} = 8.7 \text{ in.}^2$

19. **A)**

The mean is equal to the sum of the results divided by the number of results:

$\dfrac{1+3+5+x}{4} = 2.5$

$1 + 3 + 5 + x = 10$

$x = 1$

20. **C)**

To find the mean, divide the sum of the data points by the number of data points:

Mean of seventh graders $= \dfrac{2+1+1+2+2}{5}$

$= 1.6$

Mean of tenth graders $= \dfrac{0+1+1+0}{4} = 0.5$

Now find the difference:

$1.6 - 0.5 = 1.1$

21. **B)**

Divide the percentage who enrolled at a small public university by the total percentage who enrolled in a public university:

$\dfrac{11\%}{11\% + 38\%} = 22\%$

22. **D)**

The conversion factor of meters to feet is multiplied by 55 meters. The calculation is

$55 \text{m} \left(\dfrac{3.28 \text{ ft.}}{1 \text{ m}} \right) = 180.4 \text{ feet}$

23. **C)**

The algebraic expression can be simplified using PEMDAS:

$-(3)^2 + (5-7)^2 - 3(4-8)$

$= -(3)^2 + (-2)^2 - 3(-4)$

$= -9 + 4 - 3(-4)$

$= -9 + 4 + 12$

$= 7$

24. **D)**

The algebraic expression can be simplified using PEMDAS:

$(3^2 \div 1^3) - (4 - 8^2) + 2^4$

$= (9 \div 1) - (4 - 64) + 16$

$= 9 - (-60) + 16$

$= 85.$

25. **B)**

The first step is to subtract (resulting in −1.88); then add the result to 14.2 (making 12.32 the solution). Line up decimal points when adding or subtracting.

26. **A)**

First, find the radius:

$r = \dfrac{d}{2}$

$r = \dfrac{5 \text{ in.}}{2} = 2.5 \text{ in.}$

Now use the formula for the volume of a cylinder:

$V = \pi r^2 h$

$V = \pi (2.5 \text{ in.})^2 (9 \text{ in.}) = 176.6 \text{ in.}^2$

27. **B)**

The least common denominator (LCD) for the three fractions is 120. To find the LCD, write each of the denominators in prime factorization form: $8 = 2^3$, $10 = 2 \times 5$, $3 = 3 \times 1$. The least common multiple of 8, 10, and 3 is the product of all the prime numbers in these factorizations to their highest power. So the LCD $= 2^3 \times 3 \times 5 = 120$.

To write each fraction in equivalent form with a denominator of 120, the first fraction is multiplied by $\frac{15}{15}$, the second fraction is multiplied by $\frac{12}{12}$, and the third fraction is multiplied by $\frac{40}{40}$. The problem is now:

$\frac{105}{120} - \frac{12}{120} - \frac{80}{120} = \frac{93}{120} - \frac{80}{120} = \frac{13}{120}$

28. **D)**

The fraction $\frac{10}{11}$ is changed to a decimal by long dividing 11 into 10 with the result of 0.909090... Therefore, the solution is $4.\overline{90}$ since the decimal repeats.

29. **A)**

The digit in the hundreds place is 3. It is rounded up to 4 because the digit in the tens place is 6, which is greater than or equal to 5. The number is thus rounded up to 74,400. The digit in the thousands place is 4, and remains 4 because the digit in the hundreds place (3) is less than 5. The number is therefore rounded to 74,000.

30. **C)**

The total amount of sales for the week is $2,700. The lowest amount of sales was on Tuesday and the largest was on Saturday. The ratio for Tuesday is $\frac{250}{2700} = \frac{5}{54}$ and the ratio for Saturday is $\frac{800}{2700} = \frac{8}{27}$.

31. **B)**

Start by combining like terms on each side:

$8y - 8 = 9y - 22$

Next, subtract $8y$ from both sides:

$8y - 8 - 8y = 9y - 22 - 8y$

$-8 = y - 22$

Finally, add 22 to both sides:

$-8 + 22 = y - 22 + 22$

$y = 14$

32. **B)**

Changing a percent to a decimal requires that the decimal point be moved two places to the left. Moving the decimal in 37.5 to the left two places results in 0.375.

33. **D)**

The first step is to find the amount of change by multiplying 37,500 by 0.055 (5.5% written as a decimal), which is $2,062.50. The amount of change, added to the original salary, is $39,562.50.

Alternatively, recognize the fact that the employee is now earning 105.5% of what he or she earned before. Calculate the new salary by multiplying 1.055 × 37,500 = 39,562.50.

34. **D)**

The values are easily compared if all are written in decimal form. The decimal values for D are

$-1.1, -0.8, -0.13, 0.7,$ and $.\overline{81}$. This is the only answer choice listed from least to greatest.

35. **C)**

The percent of change is the amount of change divided by the original amount, multiplied by 100. The amount of change is 7375 – 7250 = 125. The percent change is $\frac{125}{7250} \times 100 = 1.7\%$.

36. **B)**

Since all the numerators are the same, the numbers can be ordered by comparing the denominators. The largest positive fractions have the smallest denominators (since dividing by larger numbers creates smaller fractions). For the negative fractions, the fraction closest to 0 (and therefore the largest) will be the one with the smallest absolute value (and largest denominator). Alternately, each of the fractions can be changed to decimals as $0.\overline{3}, -0.25, 0.5, -0.2, 0.\overline{142857}, -0.1\overline{6}$. The fractions written in order from greatest to least are $\frac{1}{2}, \frac{1}{3}, \frac{1}{7}, -\frac{1}{6}, -\frac{1}{5}, -\frac{1}{4}$.

Reading

1. **D) is correct.** The passage describes human studies as the study of "the relationship between human activity and the environment," which would include farmers interacting with river systems.

2. **A) is correct.** The passage explains what the study of geography involves and outlines its main sub-disciplines.

3. **B) is correct.** Only this choice summarizes the two main points of the passage: the definition of geography and the breakdown of its sub-disciplines.

4. **A) is correct.** The raffle is the only feature described as an event the organizers will be "bringing back."

5. **C) is correct.** The "record number of visitors" is the highest, or best, number of visitors to the fair.

6. **C) is correct.** The passage is trying to persuade people to attend the Friendswood Village Summer Fair.

7. **A) is correct.** Only "Facial Expressions" fits with the other subheadings under the category "Involuntary Physical Symptoms of Emotion."

8. **A) is correct.** Page 155 is included in the section that covers the end of World War II.

9. **C) is correct.** Page 311 is included in the section on depictions of the Cold War in popular culture between 1945 and 1991.

10. **B) is correct.** The author notes de Tocqueville's observation: "The more I advanced in the study of American society, the more I perceived that the equality of conditions is the fundamental fact from which all others seem to be derived," implying that equality was the most important ideal in the United States.

11. **A) is correct.** *New* best describes the idea that the writer is encountering things he has never seen before.

12. **D) is correct.** "Equality of conditions" suggests that people's living conditions, in terms of economics and social status, were equal.

13. **B) is correct.** Letters from a first-hand witness would be a primary source.

14. **B) is correct.** The word *conquistadors* is italicized to indicate it is in a foreign language.

15. **A) is correct.** Only *Green Tea* fits the pattern of headings that describe categories of tea based on color.

16. **B) is correct.** The fact that the light is affecting how a painting is viewed implies that the word light is being used to describe the electromagnetic waves that make human vision possible.

17. **C) is correct.** Of the four choices, only Sycamore Apartments is located on Main Street south of the train station.

18. **B) is correct.** The scale shows that the two buildings are approximately 1 mile apart.

19. **D) is correct.** This choice lists the steps for brewing coffee in the same order as the passage.

20. **A) is correct.** The author describes the steps for making coffee in chronological order.

21. **B) is correct.** The writer uses the first person, showing his or her opinion, to recommend a French press as the best way to brew coffee.

22. **D) is correct.** The passage mentions several times that decisions about things like water minerals, ground size, and steep time will depend on the preference of the coffee drinker.

23. **A) is correct.** The passage as a whole describes from start to finish how to make a cup of coffee the drinker will enjoy.

24. **A) is correct.** The author argues that "every man, woman and child should learn" to swim, and then explains to the reader why he or she should be able to swim.

25. **D) is correct.** The author wants to persuade the reader that swimming is a necessary skill.

26. **B) is correct.** As shown in the title and opening sentence, the passage is written to inform students about changes to the policy.

29. **C) is correct.** *Misuse* best describes the passage's implication that student ID cards have been used incorrectly or fraudulently.

28. **B) is correct.** The new policy states that the "student must apply for a replacement ID card in person at the Student Admissions Office. Online applications will no longer be accepted."

29. **B) is correct.** The passage is narrative, meaning it tells a story.

30. **C) is correct.** The crowd's support for Alfie and their collective roar after the shot implies that Alfie scored the goal and won the championship.

31. **C) is correct.** The metaphor implies that Alfie felt pressure from the people watching him to perform well. There is no indication that he is threatened physically.

32. **D) is correct.** This statement starts with the phrase *to begin*, which introduces a series or sequence.

33. **A) is correct.** Choice A shows the correct order and placement of the triangles after following the directions.

34. **D) is correct.** While the passage opens with a congratulatory message, the main purpose of the passage is to ask for a list of job responsibilities and training materials from Hannah.

35. **B) is correct.** The tone and content of the passage implies that the writer is a coworker of Hannah's. She is likely not her manager, since she just learned of the promotion. She is also not the replacement, since she is planning to train that person in the future.

36. **B) is correct.** The passage states that 402 students went on to attend college or university, and 11 percent of 402 is approximately 44 students.

37. **A) is correct.** The passage is written in a neutral, professional tone. It does not include any informal, emotional, or first-person language.

38. **D) is correct.** Only this recipe does not include milk or butter, both of which are dairy products.

39. **D) is correct.** The passage gives a short history of thermonuclear weapons and then introduces its main topic—the physical and biological consequences of nuclear war.

40. **B) is correct.** The main purpose of the passage is to inform customers about the accounting error and to let them know how they will receive their refunds.

41. **C) is correct.** The company ends the passage by expressing its appreciation for customers and offering both a discount and a personal contact within the company, implying it is trying to improve customer relations.

42. **C) is correct.** The index shows that page 135 is the first mention of Norway in the book.

43. **A) is correct.** The index shows that page 15 is the first mention of Niger in the book.

44. **A) is correct.** The bulk of the passage is dedicated to showing that conventional wisdom about "fewer calories in than calories out" isn't true for many people and is more complicated than previously believed.

45. **C) is correct.** The author cites several scientific studies to support the argument.

46. **D) is correct.** People misreporting the amount of food they ate would introduce error into studies on weight loss and might make the studies the author cites unreliable.

47. **B) is correct.** Paper Clips & Staples offers the cheapest shipping and handling cost for a 22-pound package.

48. **C) is correct.** Quick & Fast Office Supplies offers the cheapest shipping and handling cost for an 11-pound package: 7.99 + (1.99 × 1) = $9.98.

49. **A) is correct.** The passage states that "the best time to remove the roots, and take away the offsets, is in August."

50. **B) is correct.** *Multiplied* best describes the passage's description of how the plant reproduces by producing offsets.

51. **C) is correct.** The figure shows that pyrimidines have a single carbon nitrogen ring, while purines have two.

52. **C) is correct.** 12 degrees F (Fahrenheit) corresponds to 54 degrees C (Celsius) on the thermometer's scale.

53. **A) is correct.** The stomach is the only choice that is an organ in the human digestive tract.

Science

1. **B) is correct.** Internal respiration is the process that occurs after oxygen leaves the lungs via the alveoli.

2. **B) is correct.** Sebum is secreted by the sebaceous glands in order to coat and prevent hair and skin from drying.

3. **D) is correct.** Ligaments are made of flexible collagen fibers and play a key role in joint movement and bone stabilization.

4. **D) is correct.** Uracil (U) is a pyrimidine found in RNA, replacing the thymine (T) pyrimidine found in DNA.

5. **C) is correct.** Keratin, produced by keratinocytes, makes up the majority of the epidermis structure, hair, and nails.

6. **D) is correct.** The atomic number is the number of protons in an atom and defines the type of atom. Elements are arranged on the periodic table in order of increasing atomic number.

7. **A) is correct.** Scientific laws, like Newton's laws of gravity or Mendel's laws of heredity, describe phenomena in the natural world that have repeatedly occurred with no known exceptions yet.

8. **C) is correct.** Red blood cells contain hemoglobin, which is a molecule that transports oxygen.

9. **D) is correct.** Hormones are considered chemical mediators of the endocrine system and depend on the circulatory system for distribution. They elicit responses by binding to cellular receptors at the targeted tissues.

10. **D) is correct.** Nails, not hair, help protect soft tissue from injury.

11. **A) is correct.** Cytoplasm breaks down material that enters through the cell membrane.

12. **A) is correct.** Abduction occurs when muscles contract and move a body part away from the midline; the muscle completing this movement is called an abductor muscle.

13. **D) is correct.** Both qualitative and quantitative methods must be held to the same standard of scientific rigor.

14. **B) is correct.** A vascular nevis, or hemangioma, is a red-colored birthmark caused by a proliferation of blood vessels.

15. **A) is correct.** The valence shell is the electron orbital shell that is furthest from the nucleus and incompletely filled.

16. **A) is correct.** Muscles contract and exert force on the bone, working in tandem to create movement.

17. **A) is correct.** The cell cycle consists of three stages: interphase, or cell growth; mitosis, the division of chromosomes and nucleus; and cytokinesis, the division of the cytoplasm.

18. **C) is correct.** Allergies occur when the immune system treats a common foreign substance as a pathogen and attacks the substance with the IgE antibody.

19. **D) is correct.** The diaphragm is a muscle that increases the thoracic cavity when contracted, allowing more space for the lungs during respiration.

20. **B) is correct.** All white blood cells begin to develop in bone marrow; some of these cells mature in the bone marrow and are called B cells.

21. **B) is correct.** A heterozygous gene contains two alleles that are different from one another; one will be expressed as the dominant allele in the phenotype.

22. **B) is correct.** As actin and myosin molecules in muscle bands slide past one another, they pull the opposite ends of the cell toward one another and create contraction by shortening the length of the muscle.

23. **A) is correct.** London dispersion forces arise due to the random movement of electrons and may be found in all atoms and molecules.

24. **A) is correct.** Steroids are a type of cholesterol-derived hormone.

25. **B) is correct.** Phagocytosis is an important innate immune response to pathogens, in which foreign bodies are ingested and destroyed by phagocytic cells.

26. **D) is correct.** Correlation is a measure of the relationship between two variables; causation only exists if one variable (cause) impacts the other (effect).

27. **A) is correct.** Alveoli are sacs at the end of the respiratory tree in the lungs and are the area of gas exchange.

28. **A) is correct.** The seminal vesicles provide nourishment for sperm and up to 70 percent of the total volume of semen.

29. **C) is correct.** The celiac artery is the first and largest branch of the abdominal aorta and supplies oxygenated blood to the stomach, spleen, liver, and esophagus.

30. **D) is correct.** Fertilization does not occur until after sperm has fully matured and been released to an egg.

31. **D) is correct.** Blood is metabolized by liver cells in the sinusoidal capillaries before exiting the liver via the hepatic vein.

32. **A) is correct.** A heterogeneous mixture is any non-uniform mixture, which means that the atoms or molecules are unevenly distributed.

33. **B) is correct.** Steroid hormones, such as testosterone, are lipid-soluble hormones derived from cholesterol.

34. **D) is correct.** Adaptations are features that are taken on by a population—the result of the process of evolution.

35. **A) is correct.** Plasma, the liquid portion of blood, comprises more than half of total blood volume in the average adult.

36. **D) is correct.** This statement is false; at a very high temperature, the enzyme will become denatured and will no longer be capable of catalyzing the reaction.

37. **A) is correct.** Hemoglobin in red blood cells binds to oxygen molecules and transports them from the lungs throughout the body.

38. **A) is correct.** All experiments involving humans must use only willing volunteers; scientists must never coerce unwilling subjects. This ethical consideration is unrelated to randomization.

39. **B) is correct.** The autonomic nervous system regulates involuntary functions of the heart, digestive tract, and other smooth muscles; it is further subdivided into the sympathetic and parasympathetic nervous systems.

40. **A) is correct.** Neurons typically have one long, thick axon that transmits signals away from the neuron.

41. **B) is correct.** An action potential is the quick rise and fall of the electrical potential in a neuron.

42. **D) is correct.** The cerebrum, cerebellum, and brain stem are considered the three major portions of the brain; all brain regions are found within these three portions.

43. **C) is correct.** A catalyst makes it possible for a reaction to proceed by an alternative route, thus lowering the activation energy and speeding up the reaction.

44. **B) is correct.** Both urine and semen travel through the penile urethra, the longest portion of the male urethra, to be expelled through the urethral opening.

45. **B) is correct.** The rib cage, which consists of the ribs and the sternum, is part of the axial skeleton.

46. **D) is correct.** The independent variable is changed by the researcher during an experiment; this change may or may not cause a direct change in the dependent variable.

47. **D) is correct.** The five lumbar vertebrae are found in the lower back where the spine curves down toward the abdomen.

48. **C) is correct.** A null hypothesis assumes that any relationship is due to chance.

49. **C) is correct.** External validity can be further divided into two types: population validity, a measure of how applicable conclusions are to a population, and ecological validity, a measure of how much the situation impacts the experiment results.

50. **C) is correct.** All muscle tissues are considered soft tissue; therefore, soft muscle is not considered a separate type of muscle in the human body.

51. **C) is correct.** The epididymis is a coiled tube that receives spermatozoa and stores them for up to three months before transporting them to the vas deferens.

52. **A) is correct.** Fat-soluble, or lipophilic, hormones pass through cell membranes to attach to receptors. The receptors then bind to DNA to activate the targeted gene.

53. **B) is correct.** This is an example of human error, or error that occurs when the researcher makes a mistake.

English and Language Arts

1. **C) is correct.** The titles of musicals are always italicized.

2. **C) is correct.** *Presidential* is an adjective describing the election and, as such, should not be capitalized.

3. **B) is correct.** The text following the explanation elaborates on what was said in the first part of the sentence, and is not an independent clause, so a colon is needed.

4. **C) is correct.** Subject and verb only agree in Choice C. In Choice A, *Garden* requires a singular verb (*offers*), as does *System* in Choice B (*is*). In Choice D, the subject *field* requires a singular verb (*is*).

5. **B) is correct.** Choice B is written in an academic style. Choice A discusses a topic that isn't relevant to a scientific paper. Choice C inappropriately uses the first person, and Choice D uses informal language (*really silly*).

6. **A) is correct.** The predicate includes the main verb of the sentence.

7. **D) is correct.** *Interupted* should be spelled *interrupted*.

8. **B) is correct.** *Enviornmentalists* should be spelled *environmentalists*.

9. **C) is correct.** *Normalized* best describes the idea the bats are now all the same shape, size, and weight.

10. **C) is correct.** The prefix *anti–* means *opposite* or *against*. *Fore–* means *before*, *bi–* means *two*, and *trans–* means *across*.

11. **D) is correct.** *Each of which* is singular, so it requires the singular pronoun *its*.

12. **B) is correct.** *Disrespectful* best describes the idea that the students were behaving rudely and deserved to be disciplined.

13. **C) is correct.** *Chron* is used in words relating to time (e.g., *chronology*, *synchronize*).

14. **D) is correct.** Here, a comma correctly sets off the introductory phrase; furthermore, the sentence does not include an apostrophe in the pronoun *its*.

15. **A) is correct.** The first clause is dependent and the second is independent, so they should be joined by a comma.

16. **A) is correct.** *Improving* best conveys the idea described in the sentence that Esperanto was intended to enhance international communication.

17. **D) is correct.** Only Choice D includes a single independent clause with no other clauses.

18. **B) is correct.** The prefix *lexi–* means *related to words*.

19. **D) is correct.** An independent clause (*the fully…of Rome*) is connected with a dependent clause (*Although organized…Egyptian times*) using a comma.

20. **A) is correct.** The other choices all discuss the importance of the game to the town, so Choice A does not belong.

21. **C) is correct.** In the sentence, *handsome* is an adjective describing Narcissus.

22. **D) is correct.** In the sentence, *drag* is used as a slang term that means something is annoying or boring.

23. **A) is correct.** The comma is not needed to separate *such as* from the list it introduces. A comma is needed to separate items in a series (Choice B) and to set apart an introductory phrase (Choice C). The sentence does not

convey emotion or ask a question, so a period (Choice D) is appropriate.

24. **A) is correct.** *Shelf* is correctly made plural as *shelves*. *Phenomenons* should be *phenomena*, *mans* should be *men*, and *deers* should be *deer*.

25. **B) is correct.** *Travels* functions as a noun and is the subject of the sentence.

26. **A) is correct.** A comma should never separate a subject (*Nile River*) from its verb (*passes*). Choice B correctly separates the dependent from the independent clause. Choice D correctly ends the sentence.

27. **D) is correct.** Only in this choice do the three phrases have a similar (parallel) structure (verb + direct object).

28. **C) is correct.** The outline shows that the First Stage of labor is broken down into three phases (Early, Active, and Transition).

Made in the USA
San Bernardino, CA
30 November 2016